Holistic Liver Healing Bible

The Fatty Liver Fix

A Science-Based 30-Day Protocol to Cleanse, Repair, and Restore Your Liver for Lasting Energy and Optimal Digestive Health

GRAPEVINE BOOKS

Published by

GRAPEVINE BOOKS

www.grapevinebooks.com

email: contact@grapevinebooks.com

Ordering Information:

Quantity sales: Special discounts are available on quantity purchases by corporations, associations, and others.

For details, reach out to the publisher.

First published by Grapevine Books, 2025

Contents

Get Your Free E-book

Get Your Free E-book
Scan the QR code below to instantly access the
e-book ' **The Liver-Cleanse Pantry**', absolutely free

SCAN ME

https://bonus.grapevinebooks.com/livercleansepantry

Part 1

Understanding Your Liver: The Foundation of Health

Chapter 1: The Liver's Role in Your Health

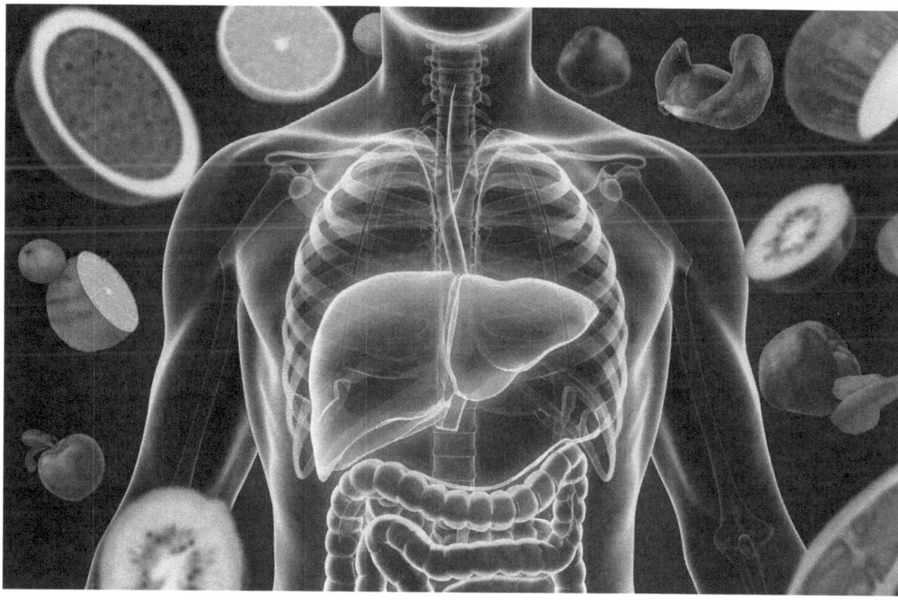

The liver is the only solid organ in the human body with the remarkable ability to regenerate itself after injury. Even if up to 70 percent of the liver is damaged or removed, it can grow back to its original size and restore function in a matter of weeks. This is not a random biological accident. It is a carefully designed survival mechanism that protects you from long-term damage caused by toxins, infections, and daily metabolic waste.

1. Why the Liver is the Body's Master Regenerator

Key regenerative abilities of the liver:

- **Cellular renewal**: Liver cells, or hepatocytes, can multiply rapidly to replace damaged tissue.
- **Toxin filtration reset**: As the liver heals, it restores its full detoxification capacity.
- **Nutrient processing recovery**: Regeneration ensures that digestion, blood sugar regulation, and nutrient storage return to normal.

Why this matters for you:

When you understand that the liver is not static but dynamic, you realize that past damage is not a life sentence. With the right conditions, your liver can recover. This ability is what makes early intervention for fatty liver disease, inflammation, or chemical exposure so effective.

2. The Liver's Role in Detoxification, Digestion, and Metabolism

The liver is the command center for several critical functions that keep you alive and healthy. To appreciate how central it is to your well-being, you need to understand the three major roles it plays.

1. Detoxification

Every day, your liver filters your blood, removing harmful substances such as:

- Metabolic waste products like ammonia
- Environmental toxins such as pesticides and heavy metals
- By-products from alcohol and medication processing

The detox process happens in two main phases:

1. **Phase One**: Converts toxins into intermediate substances.
2. **Phase Two**: Binds these substances with other molecules to make them water-soluble for elimination through urine or bile.

A poorly functioning liver means toxins accumulate, which can lead to symptoms such as fatigue, brain fog, skin issues, and hormonal imbalances.

2. Digestion

The liver produces bile, a fluid essential for breaking down fats and absorbing fat-soluble vitamins such as A, D, E, and K.

Functions of bile:

- Emulsifies fats into smaller particles for easier digestion
- Helps the intestines absorb nutrients
- Supports elimination of waste products through stool

Without healthy bile production, even a perfect diet can leave you undernourished.

3. Metabolism

The liver is a central hub for managing energy balance. It regulates blood sugar levels, stores glycogen for quick energy, and processes amino acids from protein.

Metabolic functions include:

- **Blood sugar regulation**: Prevents extreme highs and lows.
- **Fat processing**: Converts excess carbohydrates into fatty acids for storage, but also breaks them down when needed for energy.
- **Protein metabolism**: Produces proteins needed for blood clotting and immune function.

If liver metabolism slows, it can lead to weight gain, sluggishness, and reduced resilience to illness.

3. The Liver–Gut Connection and Whole-Body Wellness

Your liver does not work alone. It forms a close partnership with your digestive system, particularly the gut microbiome. This gut-liver axis plays a crucial role in both health and disease.

The Gut-Liver Axis Explained

Nutrients, toxins, and bacterial by-products from your digestive tract travel to the liver through the portal vein. The liver processes and filters these substances before they enter general circulation.

Why this matters:

- If the gut microbiome is healthy, the liver receives fewer toxins and inflammatory compounds.
- If the gut is imbalanced, harmful substances can overwhelm the liver's detox systems.

Impacts on Immunity

The liver is also part of your immune defense. Specialized immune cells called Kupffer cells patrol for pathogens in the blood. If gut health is poor, the immune system in the liver is constantly under stress, which can trigger inflammation and contribute to liver diseases such as non-alcoholic fatty liver disease.

Gut Health and Hormones

The gut-liver connection also affects hormonal balance. A healthy gut helps the liver metabolize and eliminate excess hormones, while an unhealthy gut can cause hormonal buildup that affects mood, energy, and weight.

Practical Insights for Protecting the Liver–Gut Partnership

While later chapters will go into detailed dietary and lifestyle strategies, you can start protecting this connection with three simple principles:

1. **Eat a variety of fiber-rich foods**: This supports beneficial bacteria that reduce toxin load.
2. **Stay hydrated**: Water aids both bile production and toxin elimination.
3. **Limit ultra-processed foods**: These often contain additives and excess sugars that strain both the gut and the liver.

A Partnership That Shapes Health

Your liver and gut are in constant conversation. Every meal you eat, every drink you sip, and every supplement you take is processed through this partnership. The gut breaks down food, and the liver processes nutrients, removes harmful compounds, and prepares the body for optimal energy use.

This is called the **gut-liver axis**. It is a two-way street. If the gut is out of balance, it puts more strain on the liver. If the liver is not functioning well, it can compromise digestion and nutrient absorption. Understanding this relationship is key to preventing liver disease, improving digestion, and supporting overall vitality.

How the Gut Talks to the Liver

The two are connected through a blood vessel called the **portal vein**. This is the main route for delivering:

- Nutrients from food
- By-products of digestion
- Toxins from harmful bacteria or chemicals in food
- Signals from the gut's immune cells

When the gut is healthy, this constant stream is mostly beneficial. When the gut is imbalanced, harmful compounds slip into the bloodstream and reach the liver. Over time, this can trigger inflammation and even scarring.

When the Gut Creates Trouble for the Liver

An unhealthy gut can overload the liver in several ways:

1. **Leaky gut**
2. If the intestinal lining becomes too permeable, bacteria and toxins escape into the blood. The liver has to filter them out, increasing its workload.

3. **Unfriendly bacteria overgrowth**

4. Harmful microbes produce toxins that damage liver cells.

5. **Nutrient gaps**

6. A poor gut environment reduces nutrient absorption. Without adequate vitamins, minerals, and antioxidants, the liver struggles to repair itself.

Liver's Role in Supporting the Gut

The relationship is not one-sided. The liver also helps the gut function well by:

- **Producing bile** to break down fats and aid in nutrient absorption
- **Filtering toxins** before they can damage intestinal cells
- **Producing proteins** that regulate immune responses in the gut

If liver function drops, digestion slows, bile production falls, and gut bacteria may become imbalanced.

The Gut-Liver Axis and Inflammation

One of the most damaging outcomes of poor gut-liver communication is **chronic inflammation**. This can happen when:

- The gut sends a constant stream of toxins to the liver
- The liver is forced into overdrive to neutralize harmful compounds
- Immune cells in the liver become overactivated

Chronic inflammation not only damages liver tissue but can also affect metabolism, immunity, and brain function.

Signs That Your Gut-Liver Connection May Be Struggling

- Frequent bloating and digestive discomfort
- Unexplained fatigue after meals
- Brain fog or difficulty concentrating
- Persistent skin issues such as rashes or acne
- Irregular bowel movements
- Worsening food intolerances

Ways to Strengthen the Connection

While later chapters will offer detailed dietary protocols, here are basic steps that support both the gut and the liver:

- Eat a variety of plant-based foods to feed beneficial bacteria
- Include foods rich in prebiotic fibers such as onions, garlic, and asparagus
- Avoid excess sugar and processed oils
- Stay hydrated to aid digestion and bile flow
- Limit alcohol and unnecessary medications that strain the liver

4. How the Liver Influences Energy and Hormonal Balance

The liver is a key player in keeping your energy levels steady throughout the day. It stores and releases glucose, converts nutrients into usable fuel, and supports the breakdown of fats for long-term energy needs.

Blood Sugar Control and Energy Stability

The liver stores glucose as glycogen and releases it when your blood sugar drops. This keeps your brain, muscles, and organs supplied with energy between meals.

When liver function is impaired, blood sugar can swing too high or too low, leading to:

- Midday crashes
- Irritability when hungry
- Difficulty focusing
- Sugar cravings

Fat Metabolism for Sustained Energy

When food is scarce or during longer periods between meals, the liver converts stored fat into ketones. These ketones are an alternative energy source for the brain and muscles. If the liver is burdened by excess fat, toxins, or inflammation, this conversion slows, and your energy suffers.

The Liver as a Hormone Manager

The liver plays a quiet but vital role in regulating hormone balance. It breaks down and removes excess hormones from the bloodstream, preventing overaccumulation.

Key hormones influenced by liver function include:

- **Insulin**: Helps regulate blood sugar and fat storage

- **Estrogen**: Excess estrogen can lead to mood swings, weight gain, and menstrual irregularities
- **Cortisol**: Chronic stress can overproduce cortisol, which the liver helps clear
- **Thyroid hormones**: Needed for metabolism and energy regulation

When Hormonal Balance Slips

If the liver cannot process hormones effectively, you may notice:

- Unexplained weight gain or difficulty losing weight
- Irregular menstrual cycles or menopause symptoms
- Mood fluctuations, anxiety, or low motivation
- Sluggish metabolism even with healthy eating

Energy, Hormones, and the Inflammation Link

Chronic inflammation from poor gut-liver balance, environmental toxins, or excess liver fat can interfere with hormone signaling. This can result in:

- Insulin resistance, making blood sugar harder to control
- Increased fat storage in the liver and abdomen
- Fatigue despite adequate rest
- Reduced ability to handle stress

Everyday Practices to Support Energy and Hormonal Health

While advanced strategies appear later in the book, you can begin with:

1. **Balanced meals**: Include protein, healthy fats, and complex carbohydrates to stabilize blood sugar.
2. **Adequate sleep**: Hormone production and liver repair peak at night.
3. **Regular movement**: Gentle exercise improves insulin sensitivity and circulation.
4. **Stress management**: Deep breathing, meditation, or light stretching reduce cortisol load.
5. **Hydration**: Water helps transport nutrients and supports detox processes.

Why Energy and Hormones Depend on a Healthy Liver

Your energy is not just about calories in and calories out. Hormones dictate how your body uses fuel, and the liver is the processing plant that keeps those hormones in check. Without a healthy liver, the signals that control hunger, fat burning, and energy storage can become scrambled.

5. Early Signs of Poor Liver Health

The liver often works quietly in the background without calling attention to itself. Many people do not realize there is a problem until significant damage has occurred. Because the liver can function even when partially impaired, early symptoms may be subtle. Paying attention to these warning signs can help you take action before the condition progresses into something more serious.

Digestive and Appetite Changes

The liver plays an important role in producing bile, which helps digest fats and absorb nutrients. When its function declines, digestion suffers.

Common digestive-related warning signs:

- Persistent bloating after meals
- Nausea, especially after eating fatty foods
- Pale or clay-colored stools, indicating reduced bile flow
- Unexplained loss of appetite or aversion to certain foods
- A feeling of fullness after eating very little

Changes in Energy Levels

If the liver is not processing nutrients efficiently or is overloaded with toxins, your energy will drop.

- Ongoing fatigue that does not improve with rest
- Feeling drained after meals
- Trouble focusing or mental sluggishness
- Reduced endurance for physical activity

These signs can overlap with other conditions, but when combined with other liver-related symptoms, they deserve attention.

Skin and Eye Clues

The skin and eyes often reveal liver stress before other symptoms become obvious.

- Yellowing of the skin or whites of the eyes (jaundice) caused by elevated bilirubin

- Persistent itchiness without an apparent skin condition
- Small, visible blood vessels on the skin, sometimes called spider angiomas
- Unusual bruising or slow healing of small cuts

Hormonal and Weight Changes

Because the liver helps regulate hormones, its dysfunction can affect weight, mood, and reproductive health.

- Unexplained weight gain, especially around the abdomen
- Irregular menstrual cycles or worsening PMS symptoms
- Low libido or changes in mood such as irritability and anxiety
- Trouble losing weight despite consistent effort

Digestive Discomfort and Upper Abdominal Symptoms

Pain or discomfort in the upper right side of the abdomen can sometimes indicate liver swelling or inflammation. This may be accompanied by:

- A sense of heaviness under the ribs on the right side
- Tenderness when pressing on the area
- Occasional back pain that seems unrelated to posture or injury

Other Subtle Signs

- Persistent bad breath despite good dental hygiene
- Dark urine unrelated to dehydration
- Swelling in the legs or ankles
- Changes in sleep patterns or waking up feeling unrested

These signs by themselves do not confirm liver disease, but they are important enough to discuss with a healthcare provider, especially if multiple symptoms appear together.

6. Functional Medicine Perspective on Liver Function

Functional medicine approaches the liver not just as an organ that filters toxins, but as a key hub in an interconnected network that includes digestion, hormones, immunity, and metabolism. This perspective seeks to uncover the root causes of liver dysfunction rather than simply treating the symptoms.

Looking Beyond Blood Tests

Standard liver function tests measure markers such as ALT, AST, and bilirubin. While these can indicate damage or inflammation, they do not always reflect early-stage issues. Functional medicine practitioners may also assess:

- Nutrient status, including levels of vitamins A, D, E, K, B12, and folate
- Antioxidant capacity, particularly glutathione levels
- Inflammatory markers such as C-reactive protein
- Gut health through stool analysis
- Hormone balance including thyroid, cortisol, and sex hormones

By combining these results, a clearer picture emerges of how the liver is performing in the context of the entire body.

Root Cause Investigation

Instead of assuming a liver issue is isolated, functional medicine identifies contributing factors such as:

- **Dietary patterns** high in refined sugars, processed oils, and artificial additives
- **Chronic stress** that alters hormone balance and increases inflammation
- **Environmental toxin exposure** from cleaning products, pesticides, or plastics
- **Gut microbiome imbalances** that increase the liver's detoxification load
- **Metabolic dysfunction** such as insulin resistance or high triglycerides

This approach views the liver as a mirror reflecting overall lifestyle, environment, and metabolic health.

Supporting the Liver in Phases

Functional medicine often organizes liver support into phases that align with how the liver processes toxins.

Phase One: Preparation

- Remove harmful inputs such as alcohol, processed foods, and synthetic additives
- Support nutrient intake with antioxidant-rich fruits and vegetables

Phase Two: Optimization

- Ensure adequate protein and sulfur-rich foods like garlic, onions, and cruciferous vegetables for detoxification pathways

- Provide targeted supplements if nutrient deficiencies are detected

Phase Three: Maintenance

- Establish daily habits that reduce toxin exposure
- Continue a balanced diet that prevents the reaccumulation of liver fat and inflammation

Integration with Other Systems

Functional medicine emphasizes that liver care is inseparable from:

- **Gut health**: A healthy gut reduces toxin load on the liver
- **Hormone regulation**: Balanced hormones reduce stress on detoxification systems
- **Metabolic stability**: Controlling blood sugar helps prevent fatty liver
- **Immune health**: A strong immune system limits inflammation

This interconnectedness is why functional medicine treatments often improve multiple areas of health at the same time.

Patient Involvement and Lifestyle Design

One of the strengths of this approach is active patient participation. You are encouraged to track your own symptoms, monitor lifestyle changes, and notice how diet, stress, and sleep affect your energy and digestion.

Tools often used include:

- Food journals to identify dietary triggers
- Symptom tracking charts to measure progress
- Periodic re-testing of liver markers and nutrient levels
- Goal setting for sustainable habit changes

Practical Everyday Steps from the Functional Medicine Approach

While a customized plan is best created with a practitioner, general principles include:

- Eating a variety of whole, minimally processed foods
- Avoiding unnecessary medication unless prescribed for a clear medical reason
- Prioritizing restorative sleep and stress-reducing activities

- Staying physically active without overexertion
- Using filtered water to limit chemical intake
- Reducing exposure to household and environmental toxins

Functional medicine does not see liver health as a separate project but as part of a larger goal of restoring balance to the body. By identifying the connections between the liver and other systems, this approach can prevent recurring issues and create a long-term path to wellness.

Chapter 2: Common Liver Conditions and Warning Signs

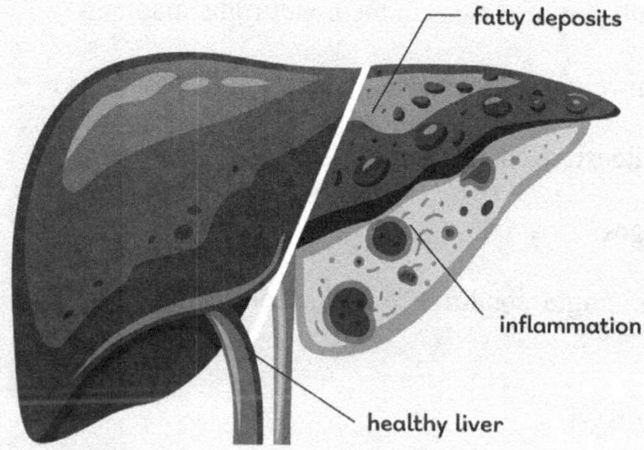

1. Fatty Liver (NAFLD) Causes, Symptoms, and Stages of Progression

Non-alcoholic fatty liver disease, often shortened to NAFLD, refers to the buildup of excess fat in liver cells in people who drink little or no alcohol. A healthy liver contains some fat, but when fat makes up more than five to ten percent of its weight, it is considered fatty liver. NAFLD is now one of the most common liver conditions worldwide, affecting adults, teenagers, and even children.

Primary Causes

NAFLD develops gradually and often reflects the influence of multiple factors.

- Diets high in refined carbohydrates and added sugars
- Excess caloric intake leading to weight gain
- Insulin resistance and metabolic syndrome
- Sedentary lifestyle with low muscle activity
- High triglyceride and cholesterol levels
- Certain medications that affect fat metabolism
- Poor gut health contributing to inflammation and toxin overload

Symptoms to Watch For

Early stages of NAFLD rarely cause discomfort. Many people only discover it after a routine blood test or imaging scan. However, some symptoms may develop:

- Persistent fatigue
- Mild discomfort or heaviness in the upper right abdomen
- Unexplained weight gain, especially around the midsection
- Occasional digestive changes, such as bloating or nausea

Progression Stages

NAFLD is not a single condition but a spectrum that can worsen over time if left unchecked.

1. **Simple fatty liver**
   - Fat accumulates in liver cells, but there is little to no inflammation or scarring.
   - Often reversible with lifestyle changes.
2. **Non-alcoholic steatohepatitis (NASH)**
   - Fat buildup is accompanied by inflammation and liver cell injury.
   - Can lead to fibrosis (scarring).
3. **Fibrosis**
   - Scar tissue begins to form in response to ongoing inflammation.
   - The liver still functions, but with reduced efficiency.
4. **Cirrhosis**
   - Extensive scarring replaces healthy tissue.
   - Liver function declines significantly and complications increase.

2. Non-Alcoholic Steatohepatitis (NASH) and Its Risks

What is NASH

NASH is a more aggressive form of fatty liver disease. It occurs when fat accumulation in the liver is accompanied by significant inflammation and cell damage. This ongoing injury stimulates the formation of scar tissue, which can spread if the underlying causes are not addressed.

Who is Most at Risk

- People with obesity, especially abdominal fat
- Those with type 2 diabetes or prediabetes
- Individuals with high blood pressure or abnormal cholesterol levels
- People with a family history of liver disease
- Those exposed to certain environmental toxins or long-term medications

How NASH Differs from NAFLD

While all NASH cases begin with fat accumulation, not all cases of NAFLD progress to NASH. The difference lies in the presence of:

- Significant inflammation within the liver
- Ongoing liver cell damage visible under a microscope
- Higher likelihood of developing fibrosis and cirrhosis

Symptoms of NASH

In many cases, symptoms are subtle or absent until later stages. Potential signs include:

- Persistent upper right abdominal discomfort
- Ongoing fatigue not relieved by rest
- Unexplained weight changes
- Mild swelling in the legs or abdomen due to fluid retention

Complications if Untreated

NASH can lead to:

- Progressive fibrosis and cirrhosis
- Increased risk of liver cancer (hepatocellular carcinoma)
- Higher likelihood of needing a liver transplant
- Greater cardiovascular risk due to systemic inflammation

Standard blood tests cannot always distinguish between simple fatty liver and NASH. Diagnosis often requires imaging studies, and in some cases, a liver biopsy to confirm inflammation and scarring.

3. Hepatitis, Cirrhosis, and Other Liver Diseases

Hepatitis is inflammation of the liver, most often caused by viral infections, but also linked to toxins, autoimmune conditions, and alcohol use.

Major types of viral hepatitis include:

- **Hepatitis A**

Spread through contaminated food or water. Usually short-term and self-limiting, but can be serious in vulnerable individuals.

- **Hepatitis B**

Spread through blood, sexual contact, or from mother to child during birth. Can become chronic and lead to liver damage.

- **Hepatitis C**

Transmitted mainly through blood-to-blood contact. Often becomes chronic and is a major cause of cirrhosis and liver cancer.

- **Hepatitis D and E**

Less common but can cause severe illness in certain settings.

Cirrhosis

Cirrhosis is the result of long-term liver damage where healthy tissue is replaced with scar tissue. This scarring prevents the liver from functioning normally and can cause:

- Jaundice
- Swelling in the abdomen (ascites)
- Confusion due to toxin buildup in the brain (hepatic encephalopathy)
- Easy bruising and bleeding
- Severe fatigue

Causes of cirrhosis include:

- Chronic hepatitis B or C
- Long-standing NASH or alcoholic liver disease
- Certain genetic conditions such as hemochromatosis and Wilson's disease
- Autoimmune hepatitis

- Prolonged exposure to toxins

Other Notable Liver Conditions

- **Autoimmune hepatitis**

The immune system attacks liver cells, causing inflammation and damage.

- **Primary biliary cholangitis (PBC)**

An autoimmune condition where bile ducts in the liver are slowly destroyed.

- **Primary sclerosing cholangitis (PSC)**

Inflammation and scarring of bile ducts inside and outside the liver, often linked to inflammatory bowel disease.

- **Genetic liver diseases**

Conditions like alpha-1 antitrypsin deficiency, which impair the liver's ability to function normally.

Warning Signs to Seek Immediate Medical Help

While early symptoms may be subtle, some require urgent evaluation:

- Yellowing of the skin or eyes
- Swelling of the abdomen with sudden onset
- Vomiting blood or passing black, tarry stools
- Confusion, drowsiness, or difficulty staying alert
- Severe abdominal pain

Understanding the range of liver conditions helps identify risks before they become emergencies. Fatty liver disease, NASH, hepatitis, and cirrhosis may have different causes, but they share one truth: early recognition and proactive care can change the outcome.

4. High Liver Enzymes and What They Mean

Liver enzymes are proteins that speed up chemical reactions in the liver. When liver cells are damaged or inflamed, these enzymes can leak into the bloodstream. Routine blood tests can detect these elevated levels, which often act as an early signal that something is affecting liver health.

Key Enzymes Measured in Blood Tests

1. ALT (Alanine Aminotransferase)

Primarily found in the liver, ALT levels rise when liver cells are injured. Higher ALT readings often point to conditions like fatty liver disease, hepatitis, or certain medication effects.

2. AST (Aspartate Aminotransferase)

Found in the liver, heart, and muscles, AST can increase when there is liver damage, but it is less specific than ALT since it is present in other tissues.

3. ALP (Alkaline Phosphatase)

Present in the liver, bile ducts, and bones. Elevated ALP can suggest bile duct blockage or certain bone disorders, so context is important.

4. GGT (Gamma-Glutamyl Transferase)

Often rises with bile duct issues or excessive alcohol intake. When combined with other enzyme results, it helps pinpoint the source of the problem.

5. Bilirubin

Not an enzyme but often measured alongside them. Elevated bilirubin can lead to jaundice and signals problems with bile flow or red blood cell breakdown.

Interpreting Elevated Levels

A single abnormal reading is not always a cause for alarm. Temporary elevations can occur after intense exercise, certain medications, or even a viral illness. However, persistently high levels require investigation.

Possible Causes of High Enzymes

- Fatty liver disease (both alcoholic and non-alcoholic)
- Hepatitis infections
- Obstruction of bile ducts
- Prolonged use of certain medications such as pain relievers or statins
- Autoimmune or genetic liver disorders
- Exposure to environmental toxins

Early detection through enzyme monitoring can help identify liver stress before symptoms appear. This allows for interventions that can prevent further damage and support recovery.

5. Insulin Resistance, Triglycerides, and Liver Fat Accumulation

Insulin resistance occurs when the body's cells no longer respond effectively to insulin, the hormone responsible for moving glucose from the blood into cells. As insulin resistance increases, the pancreas produces more insulin to compensate. This imbalance has a direct impact on liver function.

How Insulin Resistance Leads to Fatty Liver

When excess glucose circulates in the bloodstream, the liver converts much of it into fat for storage. Over time, these fat deposits accumulate in liver cells, a process known as hepatic steatosis.

Step-by-step progression:

1. High sugar intake raises blood glucose levels.
2. Cells resist insulin's signals, requiring more insulin to move glucose inside.
3. The liver converts the excess glucose into fatty acids.
4. Fatty acids are stored in the liver, increasing fat content.
5. Chronic accumulation triggers inflammation and potential scarring.

The Role of Triglycerides

Triglycerides are a type of fat found in the blood. They rise when:

- Diets are high in refined carbs and sugars
- Physical activity levels are low
- Alcohol intake is excessive
- The body stores more fat than it uses

High triglycerides not only contribute to heart disease risk but also increase the likelihood of developing fatty liver disease.

Why This Combination is Dangerous

Insulin resistance, high triglycerides, and liver fat accumulation create a cycle of worsening health:

- Fat buildup impairs liver function.
- Impaired liver function makes blood sugar harder to control.
- Uncontrolled blood sugar promotes more fat storage in the liver and abdomen.

Early Indicators of This Metabolic Pattern

- Gradual weight gain, especially around the waist
- Blood test results showing elevated triglycerides or fasting glucose
- Fatigue after meals high in carbohydrates
- Cravings for sweet or starchy foods

Breaking the Cycle

Addressing all three factors together is essential. Strategies include:

- Reducing refined carbohydrates and added sugars
- Increasing physical activity to improve insulin sensitivity
- Choosing healthy fats like olive oil, nuts, and fatty fish
- Including adequate protein for blood sugar stability

6. Abdominal Bloating, Brain Fog, and Chronic Fatigue Links

Abdominal bloating, brain fog, and chronic fatigue are not just random discomforts. They often stem from underlying liver stress, gut imbalances, and systemic inflammation.

Abdominal Bloating and the Liver

When the liver struggles to produce and release bile efficiently, digestion slows. Fats may not be broken down properly, leading to gas and bloating. Additionally, if the gut microbiome is imbalanced, fermentation of undigested foods can create excess pressure and discomfort.

Possible liver-related causes of bloating include:

- Reduced bile production or flow
- Fluid retention due to early liver dysfunction
- Inflammation causing changes in gut motility

Brain Fog and Liver Function

Brain fog refers to a sense of mental cloudiness, difficulty concentrating, and slowed thinking. The liver plays a role in brain clarity because it removes toxins from the blood. If this detox process is impaired:

- Waste products can circulate longer in the body.
- Inflammatory compounds may cross into the brain.

- Energy production in brain cells may decrease.

This can result in sluggish thinking and reduced mental sharpness.

Chronic Fatigue and Energy Pathways

Fatigue linked to the liver is often different from tiredness after physical exertion. It can feel persistent and unrelated to sleep quality. This happens because:

- The liver regulates blood sugar, and unstable levels cause energy dips.
- Detoxification demands energy, leaving less available for daily activities.
- Nutrient absorption may be reduced if bile production is low.

The Overlap Between These Symptoms

When bloating, brain fog, and fatigue occur together, it often suggests:

- An overworked detoxification system
- Possible gut-liver axis imbalance
- Early signs of metabolic dysfunction

Tracking and Identifying Triggers

To understand patterns, many people keep a simple daily log noting:

- Foods eaten and timing of meals
- Onset of bloating or discomfort
- Times when brain fog appears
- Energy levels throughout the day

This can help identify connections between diet, liver stress, and symptom flares.

When to Seek Medical Evaluation

If these symptoms become persistent, it is important to discuss them with a healthcare provider. They may recommend:

- Liver function tests
- Blood sugar and triglyceride testing
- Gut health assessment
- Nutrient status evaluation

Chapter 3: Liver Tests and How to Monitor Your Progress

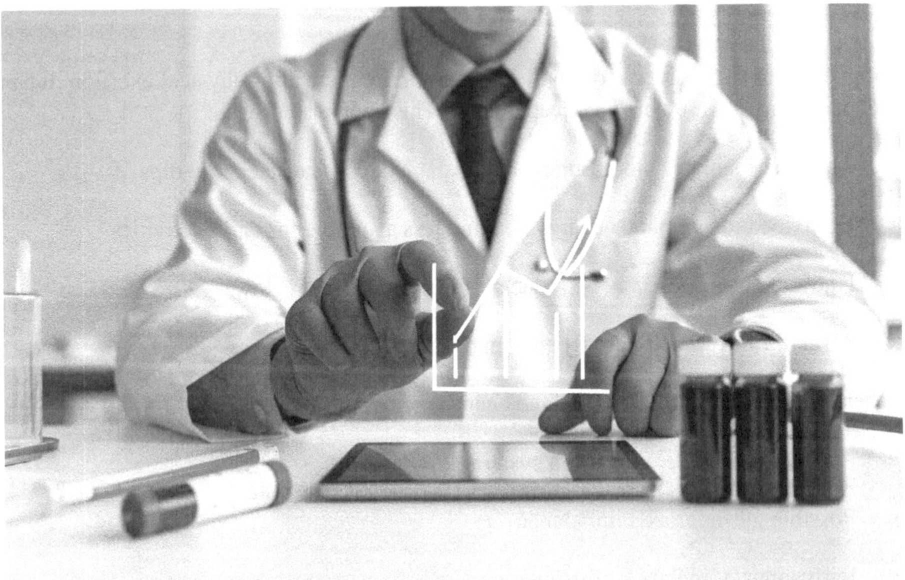

1. Understanding ALT, AST, GGT, Bilirubin, and Other Markers

Blood tests are often the first line of investigation when assessing liver health. They can reveal silent problems before symptoms appear and are also useful for tracking progress during a liver recovery program. These tests measure enzymes and other substances that reflect the liver's condition and function.

Alanine Aminotransferase (ALT)

- Primarily found in the liver.
- Elevated ALT often points to direct injury or inflammation in liver cells.
- Commonly elevated in conditions such as fatty liver disease, hepatitis, and medication-related liver stress.
- Levels usually return toward normal when the underlying cause is addressed.

Aspartate Aminotransferase (AST)

- Found in the liver but also present in muscles and the heart.
- Elevated AST can indicate liver injury, but it is not as specific as ALT.
- Comparing ALT and AST levels helps determine whether the source of the elevation is the liver or another tissue.

Gamma-Glutamyl Transferase (GGT)

- Found in liver and bile duct cells.
- A sensitive marker for bile duct problems or excessive alcohol intake.
- Often measured alongside ALP to help identify blockages or bile flow issues.

Alkaline Phosphatase (ALP)

- Found in the liver, bile ducts, and bones.
- Elevated ALP may indicate bile duct obstruction, certain liver diseases, or bone disorders.
- Interpretation requires looking at other test results and the patient's symptoms.

Bilirubin

- A yellow pigment produced when red blood cells break down.
- The liver processes bilirubin so it can be excreted through bile.
- Elevated bilirubin can lead to jaundice and signal issues with bile flow or liver function.

Other Important Markers

- **Albumin**: A protein made by the liver that helps maintain fluid balance in the blood. Low levels may indicate advanced liver disease.
- **Prothrombin Time (PT)**: Measures how long blood takes to clot. The liver produces clotting factors, so prolonged clotting time may indicate liver impairment.

How to Use These Tests for Progress Tracking

Monitoring trends over time is more important than a single reading.

- Keep a record of your test results for comparison.
- Look for consistent improvements in elevated markers as lifestyle or treatment changes take effect.
- Understand that small fluctuations are normal, but persistent high readings require attention.

2. Imaging and Non-Invasive Fatty Liver Assessments

While blood tests are useful, they cannot always tell the full story. Some people have normal enzyme levels despite having fatty liver or mild fibrosis. Imaging studies allow doctors to visualize the liver's structure, detect fat deposits, and assess the degree of scarring.

Ultrasound

- Often the first imaging test ordered for suspected liver disease.
- Uses sound waves to create images of the liver.
- Can reveal fat accumulation, changes in liver size, and some forms of scarring.
- Advantages: widely available, relatively inexpensive, and painless.
- Limitations: cannot detect very early-stage fatty liver or mild fibrosis.

FibroScan (Transient Elastography)

- A specialized test that uses ultrasound technology to measure liver stiffness.
- Stiffness often increases as fibrosis or scarring develops.
- Also estimates the amount of fat in the liver.
- Non-invasive, quick, and does not require sedation.

Magnetic Resonance Imaging (MRI)

- Provides detailed images of the liver.
- MRI with proton density fat fraction (PDFF) can accurately quantify liver fat.
- Magnetic Resonance Elastography (MRE) measures stiffness similar to FibroScan but with greater precision.
- More expensive and less available than ultrasound, but highly accurate.

CT Scan (Computed Tomography)

- Can detect moderate to severe fat accumulation.
- Not the first choice for liver evaluation due to radiation exposure.
- May be used when other imaging results are inconclusive.

Non-Invasive Scoring Systems

In addition to imaging, doctors may use scoring formulas that combine blood test results, age, and other factors to estimate the likelihood of fibrosis. Examples include:

- FIB-4 index
- NAFLD fibrosis score

These tools help determine whether further testing, such as a biopsy, is needed.

Why Avoid Jumping Straight to Biopsy

Liver biopsy is still the most accurate method for diagnosing certain liver conditions, but it is invasive and carries some risks. Most cases of fatty liver or mild fibrosis can be monitored effectively with non-invasive methods.

Tracking Your Liver Health Over Time

For anyone undergoing treatment or lifestyle changes, repeating imaging studies every 6 to 12 months can:

- Show whether fat content in the liver is decreasing
- Indicate if fibrosis is reversing, stable, or progressing
- Provide reassurance when markers and symptoms are improving

Practical Tips for Test Preparation

- Follow your doctor's instructions about fasting before blood work.
- Stay hydrated, as dehydration can sometimes affect blood test results.
- Avoid alcohol and heavy exercise in the day or two before testing, since both can temporarily raise enzyme levels.

Combining Test Results with Symptoms

Numbers and images are most useful when combined with how you feel.

- If enzyme levels drop and imaging shows improvement, but symptoms persist, further investigation is needed.
- If you feel significantly better but enzyme levels remain high, adjustments to your plan may be necessary.

3. How to Use Blood Work to Track Liver Healing Over Time

Blood work is not just for diagnosing problems. It can also serve as a map of your healing process. When you make changes to your diet, exercise habits, or supplement routine, blood tests can show whether your liver is responding positively. Interpreting these changes requires looking for trends over several months, not just reacting to single test results.

Choosing the Right Testing Schedule

For most people working to heal their liver, testing every three to six months provides enough data without becoming excessive. More frequent testing may be necessary if you have an advanced condition, are adjusting medications, or your doctor recommends closer monitoring.

Markers That Reflect Healing

The main blood markers for tracking liver recovery are often the same ones used in diagnosis, but the focus here is on their movement over time. ALT and AST should gradually move toward normal levels. ALP and GGT may decrease more slowly, but consistent downward trends are encouraging. Bilirubin levels should remain stable within the normal range.

Why Trends Matter More Than Single Results

A single test can be influenced by temporary factors such as a recent illness, physical exertion, or even dehydration. Looking at several results in sequence allows you to see the true direction of change. If liver enzymes drop steadily over three or four tests, this is a strong indication that your liver function is improving.

Context is Critical

Blood work should never be interpreted in isolation. A decrease in liver enzymes might look promising, but if you also develop other abnormal lab values, further investigation is neccssary. Similarly, a small temporary increase may not be concerning if you recently had an infection, surgery, or other stress on the body.

Communicating with Your Healthcare Provider

Ask your provider to explain the numbers in plain language and compare them to your previous results. This discussion is your chance to connect lifestyle changes with measurable effects. When you see that reducing alcohol, improving diet, or increasing exercise coincides with better blood results, motivation grows stronger.

Beyond Standard Liver Panels

In some cases, additional tests can provide a more detailed picture. These might include fasting insulin levels, hemoglobin A1c, lipid panels, or inflammatory markers such as C-reactive protein. These extra measurements can reveal improvements in related systems that affect the liver, such as blood sugar control and inflammation reduction.

Documenting Changes Over Time

Even without formal training, you can keep your own simple record of results. Note the date of each test, the key numbers, and any major lifestyle changes that happened around that time. Over the months and years, you will build a personalized history that shows your liver's journey toward recovery.

4. Home Tracking Tools and Health Journals

Why Home Tracking Matters

While blood work provides a snapshot of your liver's condition every few months, daily tracking allows you to notice subtle changes between those tests. Symptoms, energy levels, digestion, and sleep patterns can all provide clues about whether your current approach is working.

The Role of a Health Journal

A health journal is more than just a diary. It is a structured log where you record what you eat, how you feel, and any changes you make to your routine. Over time, patterns emerge that can explain why your energy improves on certain days, or why bloating returns after specific meals.

What to Record in Your Journal

A simple notebook or spreadsheet can include:

- Meals and snacks with approximate times
- Fluid intake, including water and other beverages
- Any supplements or medications
- Energy levels throughout the day
- Digestion notes such as bloating, bowel movements, or discomfort
- Sleep quality and duration
- Stress levels or emotional notes

Observing Changes in Symptoms

Not all improvements are visible in lab results right away. You might notice better digestion, reduced fatigue, or clearer skin weeks before your blood work changes. Writing these changes down ensures they are not forgotten when you meet with your healthcare provider.

Using Technology to Assist Tracking

For those who prefer digital tools, there are apps designed for health tracking. Some allow you to log meals, sleep, activity, and symptoms in one place. Others connect with wearable devices to automatically track steps, heart rate, and sleep patterns. While these tools are convenient, they should complement, not replace, your personal observations.

Tracking Specific Liver-Related Symptoms

It can be helpful to create a checklist of key symptoms to score daily or weekly. These might include:

- Energy level on a scale from 1 to 10
- Frequency and severity of bloating

- Mental clarity or brain fog
- Mood stability
- Quality of sleep

Recording these scores over time helps you see gradual shifts that might not be noticeable day to day.

Combining Home Data with Medical Results

When you bring your health journal to a doctor's appointment, you give your provider a fuller picture of what is happening between visits. This can lead to more precise recommendations and a more personalized plan. A record of consistent symptom improvement can also be encouraging when blood markers are slower to change.

Recognizing Setbacks Early

Tracking daily patterns also helps identify setbacks sooner. If energy levels drop steadily over a week, or digestive discomfort increases, you can take corrective action before the problem worsens. Early adjustments often prevent a full relapse.

Making Tracking Sustainable

The most effective tracking system is one you will actually use. For some people, that means a detailed daily log. For others, it might be a quick end-of-day note about meals and symptoms. Consistency is more important than perfection. Over time, even brief notes can build a valuable record.

The Psychological Benefit of Tracking

Recording improvements, no matter how small, reinforces your commitment. Seeing evidence that your efforts lead to better sleep, more stable energy, or reduced discomfort builds confidence that your plan is working. This positive feedback can help maintain motivation through the months of recovery.

5. What "Normal" Liver Tests Don't Always Reveal

It is common for people to receive blood test results that fall within the "normal" range yet still experience symptoms related to liver function. This happens because standard liver panels are designed to detect significant damage, not subtle or early-stage issues. The liver can lose a considerable portion of its capacity before standard tests show anything abnormal.

A reading in the normal range does not automatically mean the liver is healthy. It might only mean that the problem is not severe enough to trigger a noticeable spike in enzyme levels. Conditions such as early-stage fatty liver disease or mild bile flow issues can develop quietly while standard results remain unremarkable.

Early Dysfunction That Slips Through

Many liver conditions progress gradually. In the early stages, the body compensates well, and standard markers may stay stable. Examples include:

- Mild fat accumulation without significant inflammation
- Early bile duct narrowing or sluggish bile flow
- Low-level chronic inflammation that does not yet cause cell injury
- Minor scarring in localized areas of the liver

These situations can exist for years without crossing the threshold into abnormal results, which is why additional evaluation methods are often needed.

Why Reference Ranges Can Be Misleading

The "normal" range for a liver test is often based on statistical averages of a population, not an ideal of perfect health. In some cases, these ranges include people with undiagnosed conditions. This means a result at the high end of normal might already reflect early dysfunction. For example, someone with an ALT reading that is technically normal but higher than their historical average could be experiencing the beginning of liver stress.

The Value of Baseline Comparisons

Looking at how your numbers change over time is often more revealing than comparing them only to the standard range. A rise from an ALT of 15 to 35 within a year might still be labeled normal, yet it could indicate a shift in liver health that deserves attention. This is why keeping a personal record of past results is so valuable.

Additional Clues Beyond the Basic Panel

Sometimes, deeper testing is necessary to uncover what basic blood work misses. Specialized assessments may include:

- Tests for oxidative stress and antioxidant status
- Markers of inflammation such as C-reactive protein
- More detailed bile acid profiles
- Imaging studies to confirm or rule out structural changes

These tests can fill the gap when regular liver panels fail to match symptoms or risk factors.

Listening to the Body's Signals

Even when blood work appears fine, persistent fatigue, bloating, skin changes, or unexplained weight shifts should not be dismissed. The combination of symptoms, medical history, and lifestyle factors can reveal concerns that blood numbers alone do not capture.

6. When to Seek Medical Advice

Knowing when to consult a healthcare professional is just as important as making daily lifestyle improvements. Some symptoms and test results indicate the need for prompt evaluation, even if they seem minor. Ignoring them can allow conditions to progress to a stage where treatment is more complex.

Situations That Require Prompt Attention

- Yellowing of the skin or eyes, which may signal jaundice
- Unexplained swelling in the abdomen or legs
- Vomiting blood or passing black, tarry stools
- Confusion, disorientation, or unusual drowsiness
- Severe pain or persistent discomfort in the upper right abdomen
- Rapid and unexplained weight loss or gain

Persistent Mild Symptoms

Some warning signs are not urgent emergencies but still deserve medical review if they continue for weeks. These can include:

- Low-grade fatigue without a clear cause
- Changes in digestion, such as frequent bloating or changes in stool color
- A gradual increase in waist size despite stable eating habits
- Itchy skin without a visible rash

Acting Before the Crisis Stage

Too often, people wait until symptoms become severe before seeking help. The liver's ability to compensate for damage means that by the time pain or jaundice develops, a condition may already be advanced. Scheduling an appointment when you notice consistent, unexplained changes can allow for early intervention and simpler treatment.

Communicating Effectively with Your Healthcare Provider

When you see your doctor, bring any recent blood work, imaging results, and personal tracking notes. Clear, specific information about when symptoms began, how they have changed, and any lifestyle adjustments you have tried will help the provider make a more accurate assessment.

For example, saying "I have been more tired lately" is less useful than saying "Over the past three weeks, I have felt more fatigued in the afternoons despite sleeping seven to eight hours a night. I also noticed my appetite has decreased slightly."

The Role of Preventive Checkups

Even in the absence of symptoms, periodic medical evaluations are valuable for anyone at higher risk of liver disease. This includes people with a history of metabolic syndrome, type 2 diabetes, significant alcohol use in the past, or prolonged exposure to workplace toxins. Preventive checkups allow for early detection and create a baseline for future comparison.

Balancing Self-Monitoring and Professional Care

Tracking your own symptoms and test results at home is important, but it is not a replacement for professional evaluation. Self-monitoring helps you recognize when something changes, and professional care confirms the cause and recommends the safest path forward. The combination of both approaches offers the best protection for long-term liver health.

Acting on Intuition

Sometimes the decision to see a healthcare provider comes from a feeling that something is off, even when you cannot identify a clear reason. Trusting that instinct is wise. Subtle changes in energy, mood, or digestion can be early indicators that something is affecting your liver, even before it shows on standard tests.

Part 2

Targeted Solutions: Healing Specific Liver Problems

Chapter 4: Reversing Fatty Liver

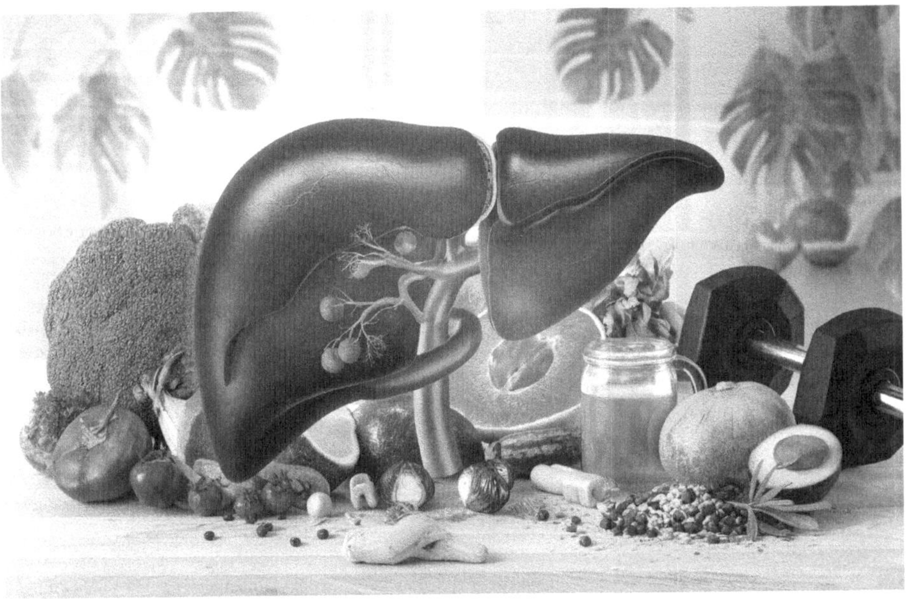

Fatty liver occurs when excessive fat builds up in the liver cells. A small amount of fat in the liver is normal, but when fat accounts for more than five percent of its weight, it begins to affect function. Over time, excess fat triggers inflammation and cellular damage. This can progress into more severe forms of liver disease if left untreated.

1. What Causes Fatty Liver and Why It's on the Rise

Dietary Changes and Modern Eating Habits

One of the biggest contributors to fatty liver is the shift in global eating patterns. Diets today often contain large amounts of refined carbohydrates, sugary beverages, processed snacks, and foods made with low-quality oils. These calorie-dense, nutrient-poor options increase fat storage in the liver.

Sedentary Lifestyles

Regular movement helps the body use stored fat for energy. When activity levels drop, the liver stores more fat. Urbanization and technology have reduced natural physical activity in daily life, which has a direct effect on liver health.

The Role of Insulin Resistance

When the body becomes less responsive to insulin, blood sugar rises. The liver attempts to manage the excess by converting glucose into fat. This fat is often stored in the liver itself, leading to hepatic steatosis.

People with type 2 diabetes or prediabetes are at significantly higher risk for developing fatty liver for this reason.

High Triglycerides and Cholesterol

Elevated blood fats are strongly linked to liver fat accumulation. A diet high in saturated fats from processed meats and fried foods, combined with low fiber intake, can cause triglycerides to rise and remain elevated.

Alcohol and Non-Alcoholic Fatty Liver

Alcoholic fatty liver is caused directly by alcohol metabolism, which stresses liver cells and promotes fat buildup. Non-alcoholic fatty liver disease (NAFLD) shares similar patterns of fat accumulation, but is driven mainly by diet, metabolism, and inflammation rather than alcohol use.

Although the causes differ, both can progress to more severe liver conditions if not addressed.

Environmental and Chemical Exposures

Certain environmental toxins, pollutants, and chemicals in household products can place an additional burden on the liver's detoxification system. When the liver is preoccupied with processing these substances, fat metabolism may slow, increasing the risk of fat buildup.

Why Fatty Liver Rates Are Increasing Globally

Fatty liver used to be associated primarily with middle-aged adults. Now, it is increasingly diagnosed in young adults and even children. This rise is linked to:

- Higher consumption of sugary drinks
- Increased portion sizes in meals
- Less daily movement and more sedentary work
- Widespread availability of processed, high-calorie foods
- Growing rates of obesity and metabolic syndrome

The combination of poor diet, lack of activity, and chronic metabolic stress has created an environment where fatty liver is more common than ever.

2. Can Fatty Liver Be Reversed? Science-Based Insights

The Liver's Regenerative Ability

The liver is one of the most resilient organs in the human body. It can repair itself by replacing damaged cells with healthy ones, provided that the source of the damage is removed. This regenerative ability means that in many cases, fatty liver can be reversed before it reaches the stage of permanent scarring.

Timeframe for Recovery

The timeline for reversal depends on the severity of the condition, overall health, and the consistency of lifestyle changes. In some individuals, measurable improvements in liver fat can be seen within weeks of dietary changes and increased activity. For others, especially those with more advanced inflammation, it may take several months or longer.

Evidence from Research

Studies consistently show that a reduction in body weight by even five to ten percent can significantly decrease fat levels in the liver. This does not always require extreme dieting; gradual, sustainable adjustments to eating habits and activity often lead to lasting results.

Research also points to the benefits of increasing fiber intake, reducing added sugars, and improving the quality of dietary fats as key strategies.

Dietary Adjustments That Support Reversal

While each person's plan will be tailored to their needs, several dietary changes have strong scientific support:

- Increasing intake of vegetables, fruits, and whole grains for fiber and antioxidants
- Replacing processed fats with healthy sources like olive oil, nuts, and fatty fish
- Reducing added sugars found in sodas, desserts, and sweetened snacks
- Eating lean protein sources such as poultry, fish, and legumes to support metabolic function
- Limiting refined grains such as white bread and pasta in favor of whole grains

Role of Physical Activity

Exercise helps reduce liver fat even without significant weight loss. Aerobic activity, such as brisk walking or cycling, improves insulin sensitivity and encourages the liver to use stored fat for energy. Strength training supports muscle mass, which increases metabolic rate and enhances fat metabolism.

Addressing Related Conditions

Reversing fatty liver is often easier when other metabolic issues are addressed at the same time. Managing blood sugar, lowering triglycerides, and reducing abdominal fat all contribute to improved liver health.

The Importance of Reducing Inflammation

Chronic inflammation not only contributes to the progression of fatty liver but also makes it harder for the liver to repair itself. Anti-inflammatory foods such as berries, leafy greens, turmeric, and green tea can help reduce this burden and create an environment that supports healing.

Sustainability Over Quick Fixes

Rapid weight loss methods or extreme cleanses may lead to temporary improvements but often come with health risks. Sustainable lifestyle changes are more effective for long-term reversal. This includes finding enjoyable forms of exercise, adopting eating habits that are realistic for daily life, and making gradual improvements rather than sudden, unsustainable shifts.

When Reversal May Not Be Fully Possible

If fatty liver has progressed to advanced fibrosis or cirrhosis, reversal becomes more difficult. In these cases, the focus shifts from removing fat entirely to preventing further damage and maintaining the best possible function. Even then, dietary and lifestyle changes can significantly improve quality of life.

Why Individualization Matters

Not all cases of fatty liver are identical. Some people may have rapid improvement with small changes, while others require more structured interventions. Genetic factors, hormonal balance, and gut health can all influence the pace and degree of recovery. This is why professional guidance, combined with personal observation, is often the most effective approach.

3. Best Diet for Reversing Fatty Liver (Foods to Eat & Avoid)

Diet is the single most influential factor in reversing fatty liver. What you eat directly affects the liver's fat content, its ability to process nutrients, and the level of inflammation inside its cells. A carefully chosen diet not only reduces fat accumulation but also improves insulin sensitivity and supports regeneration.

Unlike many restrictive plans, the best liver-healing diet focuses on abundance rather than deprivation. It prioritizes nutrient-rich foods that feed the body and protect the liver while removing items that create metabolic stress.

Foods to Prioritize

A liver-supportive diet is centered around whole, unprocessed foods that are rich in antioxidants, fiber, and healthy fats.

- **Leafy greens and cruciferous vegetables** such as kale, spinach, broccoli, and Brussels sprouts help activate detoxification pathways and are packed with anti-inflammatory compounds.
- **Berries, citrus fruits, and grapes** provide vitamin C, flavonoids, and polyphenols that reduce oxidative stress in liver cells.
- **Fatty fish** such as salmon, sardines, and mackerel supply omega-3 fatty acids that improve triglyceride levels and reduce inflammation.
- **Nuts and seeds** like almonds, walnuts, chia, and flax offer healthy fats and fiber that support metabolic health.
- **Whole grains** such as quinoa, oats, and brown rice provide steady energy without spiking blood sugar.
- **Legumes** including lentils, chickpeas, and black beans add plant-based protein and soluble fiber.

Foods to Limit or Avoid

Some foods directly contribute to liver fat accumulation and inflammation. Reducing or eliminating these items accelerates recovery.

- **Sugary drinks** including soda, fruit juices with added sugar, and sweetened teas can rapidly increase fat storage in the liver.
- **Refined carbohydrates** like white bread, pastries, and processed snack foods cause blood sugar spikes that encourage fat buildup.
- **Processed meats** such as bacon, sausage, and deli slices often contain high levels of saturated fats and preservatives.
- **Fried foods** cooked in refined oils introduce harmful compounds that stress liver cells.
- **Excessive alcohol** places a direct burden on liver detoxification and promotes fat storage.

Meal Composition and Timing

Eating balanced meals at regular intervals helps maintain stable blood sugar and reduces the chance of fat being stored in the liver. Each meal should ideally contain:

- A source of lean protein for repair and satiety
- Healthy fats to aid hormone production and nutrient absorption
- Fiber-rich vegetables for digestion and detoxification support

Spacing meals evenly and avoiding constant snacking allows the liver to process nutrients efficiently without being overwhelmed.

Making the Transition

Switching to a liver-healing diet does not have to happen overnight. Gradually replacing harmful foods with healthier options can make the changes sustainable. For example, swap soda for sparkling water with lemon, or replace refined bread with whole-grain alternatives. These shifts may seem small, but over weeks and months they create a profound impact.

4. Anti-Inflammatory Diet Principles for Liver Healing

Inflammation is a natural immune response, but when it becomes chronic, it damages tissues and slows healing. In the liver, persistent inflammation can transform simple fat buildup into more serious conditions such as fibrosis. An anti-inflammatory diet reduces this strain, creating an environment where the liver can regenerate more effectively.

Core Principles of an Anti-Inflammatory Diet

An anti-inflammatory approach is less about a rigid list of foods and more about a consistent pattern of eating that limits harmful compounds and maximizes protective nutrients.

1. Prioritize plant-based variety

Different plant foods contain unique antioxidants and phytonutrients. Eating a wide range of vegetables, fruits, herbs, and spices ensures broad coverage against oxidative stress.

2. Include healthy fats daily

Omega-3 fatty acids from fatty fish, flaxseed, chia, and walnuts help reduce inflammatory markers in the body.

3. Choose low-glycemic carbohydrates

Foods that release glucose slowly, such as sweet potatoes, lentils, and oats, help stabilize blood sugar and prevent insulin spikes that worsen inflammation.

4. Use herbs and spices strategically

Turmeric, ginger, cinnamon, and garlic have well-documented anti-inflammatory and antioxidant effects.

Minimizing Pro-Inflammatory Foods

While increasing anti-inflammatory foods is essential, limiting those that trigger inflammation is equally important. Processed oils like soybean and corn oil, excessive red meat, refined sugar, and heavily processed packaged snacks all promote inflammation and oxidative stress in the liver.

Eating for Liver-Friendly Gut Health

The gut-liver connection plays a significant role in inflammation control. Fermented foods such as sauerkraut, kimchi, and plain yogurt help support a healthy gut microbiome, which in turn reduces inflammatory compounds entering the liver. Adequate dietary fiber from vegetables, legumes, and whole grains supports this process further.

A Day on an Anti-Inflammatory Liver Diet

A sample day might include:

- Breakfast: Oatmeal with blueberries, ground flaxseed, and a sprinkle of cinnamon
- Lunch: Quinoa salad with mixed greens, chickpeas, roasted vegetables, and olive oil dressing
- Snack: A handful of walnuts and a small piece of fruit
- Dinner: Grilled salmon with steamed broccoli and sweet potato, seasoned with turmeric and black pepper

This structure balances macronutrients, provides steady energy, and delivers anti-inflammatory compounds in every meal.

Making It Sustainable

Long-term adherence is the key to success. This means choosing meals that are not only healthy but also satisfying. Experimenting with herbs, spices, and different cooking methods can keep meals flavorful while still meeting anti-inflammatory goals. Social events, travel, and busy schedules will happen, so flexibility is important. If one meal is less than ideal, returning to nutrient-rich foods at the next opportunity prevents small deviations from becoming long-term habits.

5. Supplements and Lifestyle Changes to Reduce Liver Fat

Supplements are not a replacement for diet and exercise, but they can provide targeted support when used alongside a healthy lifestyle. Certain nutrients and compounds help improve liver function, reduce inflammation, and enhance the body's ability to metabolize fat. Choosing supplements that have been studied for their effects on liver health can give an additional boost to recovery.

Nutritional Supplements with Potential Benefits

- **Omega-3 fatty acids** from fish oil or algae oil have been shown to lower triglyceride levels and improve fat metabolism.
- **Vitamin E** is a powerful antioxidant that may help reduce inflammation in people with non-alcoholic fatty liver disease, especially when combined with dietary changes.

- **N-acetyl cysteine (NAC)** supports the production of glutathione, an antioxidant the liver uses to neutralize toxins.
- **Vitamin D** deficiency is common in individuals with fatty liver, and correcting it may improve liver enzyme levels.
- **Probiotics** can help restore gut balance, which reduces the number of inflammatory compounds reaching the liver.

Cautions About Supplement Use

Even natural supplements can cause harm if taken in excess or in combination with certain medications. It is important to:

- Purchase from reputable sources that use third-party testing.
- Follow recommended dosages and avoid assuming that more is better.
- Consult a healthcare professional before starting any new supplement, particularly if you have an existing liver condition or are taking prescribed medication.

Lifestyle Adjustments that Support Fat Reduction

Supplements alone will not reverse fatty liver. Lifestyle changes create the foundation for improvement and prevent fat from re-accumulating.

Regular physical activity is a powerful tool for reducing liver fat. Both aerobic exercise and resistance training improve insulin sensitivity and encourage the body to use fat as an energy source. The key is consistency rather than intensity, especially in the beginning.

Sleep quality also plays a major role in liver health. Poor sleep increases inflammation and disrupts hormonal balance, which can promote fat storage. Aiming for seven to nine hours of restful sleep each night supports overall recovery.

Stress management is equally important. Chronic stress raises cortisol levels, which can increase blood sugar and encourage fat storage in the liver. Gentle practices such as meditation, breathing exercises, and stretching can make a noticeable difference over time.

Creating a Supportive Environment

Changing habits is easier when your surroundings match your goals. Stocking your home with liver-friendly foods, keeping workout clothes visible, and setting reminders to drink water are small but effective ways to reinforce healthy choices. Social support also matters; having friends or family members who understand your goals can help you stay consistent.

6. Herbs for Liver Repair: Milk Thistle, Turmeric, and More

Herbal medicine has been used for centuries to support the liver's detoxification and regeneration abilities. Modern research has confirmed that some herbs can protect liver cells from damage, reduce inflammation, and promote the removal of toxins. When used thoughtfully, they can complement dietary and lifestyle strategies.

Milk Thistle

Milk thistle (Silybum marianum) contains a group of compounds called silymarin, which act as antioxidants and help stabilize liver cell membranes. Silymarin is thought to protect liver cells from toxins while also encouraging the growth of new, healthy cells.

This herb is available in capsule, tablet, and tincture form. Studies suggest that milk thistle can help improve liver enzyme levels in some people with fatty liver disease, though results vary depending on the severity of the condition and overall health.

Turmeric

Turmeric contains curcumin, a compound with strong anti-inflammatory and antioxidant properties. It can help reduce liver inflammation and may improve fat metabolism. Curcumin also supports bile production, which aids digestion and the removal of waste.

Because curcumin is not easily absorbed on its own, it is often taken with black pepper extract (piperine) or consumed in whole food form alongside healthy fats.

Dandelion Root

Dandelion root has traditionally been used to stimulate bile flow and support digestion. Improved bile flow can assist in the breakdown and removal of fats, easing the liver's workload. It is available as a tea, tincture, or capsule.

Artichoke Leaf

Artichoke leaf extract may help protect liver cells and stimulate bile production. Some studies suggest it can reduce cholesterol levels and support detoxification pathways.

Schisandra Berry

Schisandra is an adaptogenic herb that has been used in traditional Chinese medicine for liver protection. It contains compounds that may improve the liver's resilience to stress and toxins.

How to Use Herbs Safely

Herbs can interact with prescription medications, so professional guidance is essential before starting any new herbal regimen. Dosage, form, and quality matter. Using standardized extracts ensures that you get consistent levels of active compounds.

It is also important to view herbs as part of a larger plan. They are not a quick fix, and their effects build gradually over weeks or months when paired with healthy food, regular exercise, and proper sleep.

Integrating Herbs into Daily Life

Some herbs can be incorporated into cooking, such as turmeric in curries or soups. Herbal teas like dandelion root or milk thistle tea provide gentle, daily support. Supplements offer more concentrated doses but should be chosen carefully.

Consistency is key. Sporadic use is unlikely to produce noticeable benefits. Setting a specific time each day to take herbal supplements or drink herbal tea can help make the habit automatic.

Chapter 5: Restoring Energy Through Liver Function

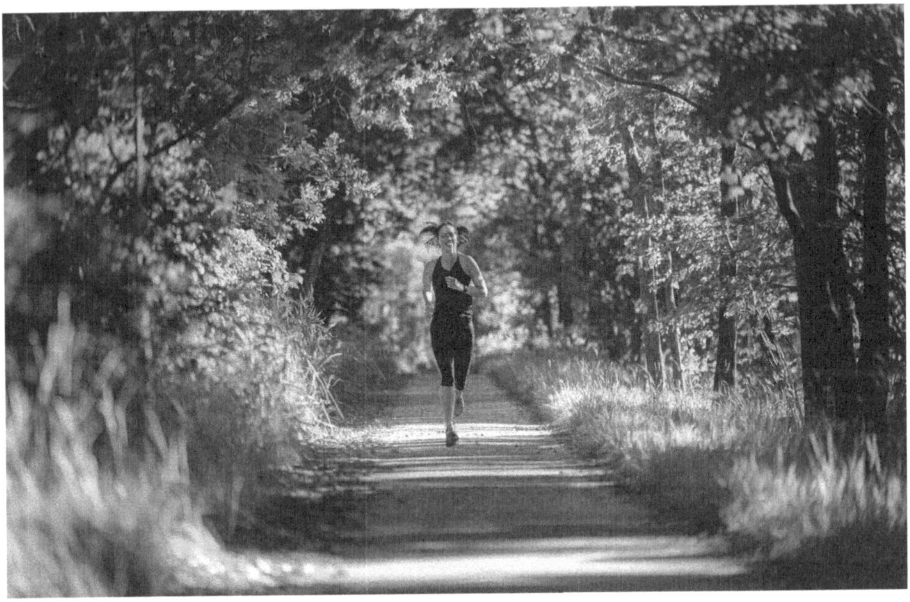

The liver is not only a detoxification organ; it is one of the body's main energy managers. It stores glucose in the form of glycogen and releases it when blood sugar drops, ensuring that the brain and muscles have a steady supply of fuel. It also converts nutrients from food into usable forms of energy and breaks down stored fat to create alternative fuel sources.

1. Why a Weak Liver Causes Fatigue and Low Energy

When the liver is stressed or damaged, these processes slow down. This means the body may struggle to maintain balanced energy levels, leading to fatigue even without significant physical exertion.

Impact on Blood Sugar Stability

A healthy liver can stabilize blood sugar levels between meals. A weakened liver, however, may release glucose irregularly, causing fluctuations that lead to feelings of tiredness or mental fog. These swings can make it difficult to focus, sustain physical activity, or maintain motivation throughout the day.

The Energy Cost of Detoxification

Detoxification requires energy. When the liver is under pressure from excess toxins, inflammation, or fat accumulation, it has to divert more resources toward processing and eliminating harmful compounds. This increased workload can leave less energy available for other bodily functions, creating a constant sense of heaviness or sluggishness.

Poor Nutrient Processing

The liver plays a major role in metabolizing proteins, fats, and carbohydrates. If it cannot perform these tasks efficiently, the body may experience nutrient shortfalls even when diet is adequate. Reduced nutrient availability directly affects mitochondrial energy production in cells, leading to persistent fatigue.

Signs That Liver Health May Be Affecting Energy

While tiredness can have many causes, the following may point toward a liver connection:

- Feeling drained shortly after eating, especially meals high in fat or sugar
- Midday crashes that improve temporarily after eating but return quickly
- General sluggishness despite a full night's sleep
- A sense of heaviness in the body during normal daily activities

The Inflammation Factor

Chronic low-grade inflammation within the liver can trigger the release of inflammatory molecules into the bloodstream. These can disrupt energy production at the cellular level and alter hormone signals that regulate metabolism. The result is not just physical fatigue but also mental and emotional exhaustion.

2. Supporting the Liver for Sustained Energy Production

Balancing Blood Sugar for Consistent Fuel

One of the most effective ways to help the liver sustain energy production is to maintain stable blood sugar levels. This can be achieved through balanced meals that combine complex carbohydrates, lean proteins, and healthy fats. Avoiding large spikes in glucose reduces the workload on the liver and ensures a steady release of fuel to the body.

Increasing Nutrient Density

Choosing foods that are high in vitamins, minerals, and antioxidants gives the liver the resources it needs to function efficiently. Nutrients like B vitamins, magnesium, and zinc are especially important for metabolic processes that convert food into usable energy. Dark leafy greens, seeds, nuts, and legumes are excellent sources.

Physical Activity to Enhance Fat Utilization

Moderate, consistent exercise encourages the liver to break down stored fat into fatty acids that can be used for energy. This process helps reduce fat accumulation in the liver while providing a reliable energy source for the body. Activities such as brisk walking, swimming, and cycling are effective without placing excessive strain on the liver.

Hydration for Optimal Function

Water is essential for the transport of nutrients and the elimination of waste. Adequate hydration supports bile production, which is necessary for fat digestion and nutrient absorption. Without enough fluids, the liver's ability to process and deliver energy to the body can decline.

Restorative Sleep

Sleep is a time for repair and regeneration. The liver is highly active during deep sleep phases, processing nutrients and removing toxins from the blood. Poor or insufficient sleep can interrupt these processes, leading to a backlog of toxins and reduced metabolic efficiency. Creating a consistent sleep routine can greatly enhance liver function and daily energy levels.

Reducing Inflammatory Load

Limiting foods and substances that contribute to inflammation helps free up liver capacity for energy production. This includes processed foods high in sugar and unhealthy fats, excessive alcohol, and unnecessary medications. Replacing these with whole, minimally processed foods supports a lower-inflammatory environment in the body.

Supporting Mitochondrial Health

The mitochondria inside cells are the actual producers of usable energy, and the liver plays a major role in supplying them with the raw materials they need. Antioxidants such as vitamin C, vitamin E, and coenzyme Q10 help protect mitochondria from oxidative stress, while adequate protein intake ensures they have the amino acids needed for repair.

Practical Daily Habits for Energy Support

While long-term strategies are essential, certain daily habits can provide immediate improvements in energy linked to liver function:

- Starting the day with a balanced breakfast containing protein and fiber
- Including a portion of fresh vegetables at every meal
- Avoiding overly large portions that place extra stress on digestion
- Taking short walking breaks during the day to keep circulation active
- Practicing stress-reduction techniques to prevent cortisol spikes that affect blood sugar

The Role of Gentle Detox Support

Gentle, ongoing detox support through foods like cruciferous vegetables, citrus fruits, and green tea can keep the liver's workload manageable. This prevents energy-draining toxin buildup while avoiding the extreme measures that can sometimes do more harm than good.

Consistency Over Intensity

Liver function improves steadily with consistent healthy choices. Sporadic bursts of intense dietary changes or exercise followed by periods of neglect do little for sustained energy. Small, regular adjustments to eating patterns, activity levels, and stress management create lasting improvements in both liver health and overall vitality.

3. Role of B Vitamins, Adaptogens, and Liver-Supportive Nutrients

B Vitamins and Energy Metabolism

B vitamins are central to how the body converts food into usable energy. The liver stores and processes several of these vitamins, releasing them as needed for metabolic reactions. When liver health declines, vitamin storage and activation can also be affected, leading to feelings of fatigue even when the diet appears adequate.

B1 (thiamine) helps break down carbohydrates into glucose, providing a quick energy source for cells. B2 (riboflavin) and B3 (niacin) play key roles in mitochondrial energy production. B5 (pantothenic acid) supports the synthesis of coenzyme A, which is necessary for fat metabolism. B6 (pyridoxine) aids in amino acid processing, while B7 (biotin) is important for glucose regulation. B9 (folate) and B12 (cobalamin) are essential for red blood cell formation, which impacts oxygen delivery and overall vitality.

Signs of Deficiency in the Context of Liver Health

When the liver struggles to store or activate B vitamins, the effects can show up as:

- Low energy and mental fatigue
- Weakness or muscle aches
- Poor stress tolerance
- Mood changes or irritability
- Slow recovery after illness or exertion

Adaptogens and Stress Support

Adaptogens are plant-based compounds that help the body adapt to stress and maintain balance. They work by influencing the hypothalamic-pituitary-adrenal (HPA) axis and moderating the release of stress hormones like cortisol. Chronic stress can harm the liver indirectly by promoting inflammation, increasing blood sugar, and altering fat metabolism.

Examples of adaptogens include:

- **Ashwagandha**, which may reduce cortisol levels and support restful sleep
- **Rhodiola rosea**, which can enhance mental clarity and reduce fatigue during stressful periods

- **Holy basil**, which may help regulate blood sugar and protect against oxidative stress

While adaptogens are not a substitute for lifestyle changes, they can help protect energy levels during recovery by supporting the body's stress response.

Other Liver-Supportive Nutrients

Several nutrients directly assist the liver's detoxification processes, antioxidant defenses, and regeneration capabilities.

- **Magnesium** is needed for hundreds of enzymatic reactions, including those related to energy production and detoxification.
- **Zinc** supports enzyme activity and helps stabilize cell membranes.
- **Selenium** is critical for antioxidant defenses and can help protect liver tissue from damage.
- **Coenzyme Q10** supports mitochondrial energy production and acts as an antioxidant.
- **Choline** aids in fat transport out of the liver, helping to prevent fatty liver buildup.

These nutrients can be obtained through a varied diet rich in vegetables, nuts, seeds, whole grains, legumes, and lean protein, but supplementation may be considered in certain cases.

Integrating Nutrients into Daily Life

It is not necessary to take every nutrient in supplement form. A well-balanced diet that includes colorful produce, a variety of protein sources, and healthy fats will naturally provide many of these compounds. Supplements should be considered only after identifying specific deficiencies or increased needs, ideally with professional guidance.

4. Detox and Energy: Finding the Right Balance

Detoxification is one of the liver's most energy-demanding tasks. Every toxin processed, every molecule of waste broken down, and every compound prepared for elimination requires metabolic fuel. If detoxification is pushed too hard or too quickly, the body may divert energy away from other functions, leading to feelings of exhaustion.

Many people experience this when they attempt extreme cleanses or rapid detox programs. While these methods can create a temporary sense of lightness, they often result in fatigue, headaches, or irritability because the body's natural systems are overloaded.

Understanding the Liver's Detox Phases

The liver detoxifies in two main stages. Phase one involves converting toxins into intermediate forms, which are often more reactive than the original substance. Phase two binds these intermediates with other molecules to make them water-soluble, allowing them to be excreted through urine or bile. Both phases require specific nutrients, antioxidants, and adequate hydration.

If phase one runs faster than phase two due to poor nutrition or insufficient support, toxins can accumulate in a more harmful state, increasing oxidative stress and contributing to fatigue.

Why Gentle, Ongoing Detox is Better Than Extreme Approaches

Supporting detoxification daily is more effective and less draining than trying to force rapid cleansing. This can be achieved by:

- Eating fiber-rich vegetables and whole grains to support elimination through the digestive tract
- Drinking enough water to aid kidney function
- Including cruciferous vegetables, citrus fruits, and herbs like parsley to support both detox phases
- Avoiding unnecessary toxin exposure from processed foods, alcohol, and environmental chemicals

Balancing Detox and Energy Preservation

While enhancing detox is important, it must not come at the cost of overall vitality. A balanced approach ensures the liver can manage its workload without compromising energy availability for muscles, brain function, and hormone balance. This means avoiding drastic calorie restriction or nutrient elimination during detox-focused phases.

Supporting the Body During Detox

During periods of increased detox activity, such as after introducing more vegetables or herbs that stimulate liver function, the body benefits from additional rest, hydration, and moderate physical activity. Light exercise like walking or stretching supports circulation without draining energy reserves. Rest allows the liver to prioritize repair and regeneration.

Listening to Energy Signals

Energy fluctuations during detox can provide valuable feedback. A mild, short-lived dip in energy may simply indicate that the liver is working harder than usual. Persistent fatigue, dizziness, or mental fog, however, can be signs that the approach is too aggressive or that key nutrients are lacking. Adjusting the pace and ensuring adequate intake of supportive foods can restore balance.

Making Detox a Sustainable Lifestyle Element

Rather than treating detox as an occasional event, it can be woven into daily living. This might mean starting the day with warm lemon water, including greens in most meals, and replacing processed snacks with fresh fruit or nuts. Over time, these habits maintain a steady detox rhythm without causing energy crashes.

5. Reversing Chronic Fatigue with Liver Support Strategies

The liver manages energy flow throughout the body by storing glycogen, regulating blood sugar, processing nutrients, and eliminating toxins. When its capacity is reduced due to fat buildup, inflammation, or nutrient shortages, fatigue can become a daily reality. This is not just a matter of feeling tired from time to time. Chronic fatigue linked to liver stress can feel persistent and overwhelming, affecting focus, mood, and physical performance.

In many cases, the body is using a significant portion of its available energy to manage ongoing detoxification and repair. This can leave less energy for daily activities, leading to that constant "running on empty" sensation.

Key Strategies to Restore Energy

Reversing chronic fatigue involves reducing the liver's workload while providing the nutrients and conditions it needs to regenerate.

- **Improve blood sugar stability** by eating balanced meals that include lean protein, healthy fats, and fiber-rich carbohydrates. This prevents rapid spikes and crashes that drain energy.
- **Support digestion and nutrient absorption** by including foods that stimulate bile flow, such as leafy greens, beets, and artichokes. Better digestion means the liver receives the raw materials it needs for energy production.
- **Lower toxin exposure** in daily life by choosing whole, minimally processed foods and reducing contact with unnecessary household chemicals. This decreases the liver's detox burden.
- **Encourage fat metabolism** through regular, moderate physical activity. Exercise prompts the liver to use stored fat as fuel, improving its efficiency and reducing excess fat accumulation.
- **Prioritize restorative sleep** to give the liver time to perform overnight detoxification and repair processes.

Addressing Inflammation to Improve Energy

Low-grade inflammation within the liver often goes hand in hand with chronic fatigue. Anti-inflammatory foods like turmeric, berries, green leafy vegetables, and omega-3-rich fish can reduce this burden. Reducing inflammation allows the liver to focus on energy-regulating tasks instead of diverting resources to damage control.

The Role of Hydration

Water is essential for optimal liver function, especially when fatigue is an issue. Adequate hydration supports the removal of waste products, keeps digestion efficient, and aids nutrient transport. Mild dehydration can magnify feelings of tiredness and sluggishness.

Building Consistency in Support Strategies

Liver recovery and the reversal of chronic fatigue require consistent effort over weeks and months. Sporadic changes are less effective. Creating a sustainable daily rhythm of supportive eating, hydration, and movement helps the body adapt gradually, leading to more lasting energy improvements.

6. Morning Rituals to Boost Energy and Metabolism

The way you start the day sets the tone for your energy and metabolism over the next several hours. The liver is highly active during the night, processing toxins, balancing hormones, and replenishing glycogen stores. Morning rituals can help the liver complete this process and prepare the body for the day ahead.

Hydration Before Caffeine

After several hours of sleep, the body is naturally in a mild state of dehydration. Drinking water soon after waking replenishes fluids, supports bile flow, and helps the liver clear out the waste products accumulated overnight. Some people find benefit in starting with warm water and lemon, which provides a gentle source of vitamin C and stimulates digestion.

A Balanced First Meal

Skipping breakfast or choosing high-sugar options can cause unstable blood sugar and sluggish energy. A breakfast that contains protein, healthy fats, and complex carbohydrates fuels the liver and maintains metabolic balance. Examples include:

- Eggs with spinach and avocado
- Oatmeal topped with berries, nuts, and a drizzle of almond butter
- Greek yogurt with chia seeds and sliced fruit

Light Movement to Wake the Body

Engaging in gentle movement in the morning improves circulation and prompts the liver to release stored energy in a controlled way. This could be stretching, yoga, a short walk, or bodyweight exercises. The goal is not intense training but rather stimulating the metabolism and helping the body transition smoothly from rest to activity.

Breathing and Mindfulness Practices

Deep breathing exercises or a few minutes of mindfulness can reduce cortisol levels, which helps prevent the mid-morning crash that often follows a stress-filled start. Lower stress in the morning also benefits the liver, as high cortisol can disrupt blood sugar balance and fat metabolism.

Supporting the Liver with Morning Nutrition

Including liver-friendly foods in the first meal of the day can provide immediate support for detox and energy processes. Leafy greens, berries, citrus fruits, and green tea supply antioxidants that help protect liver cells. Protein-rich foods provide amino acids needed for repair and regeneration.

Avoiding Morning Energy Killers

Some habits can derail energy early in the day. Consuming too much caffeine on an empty stomach can lead to jitters and later fatigue. Overly heavy breakfasts high in refined carbohydrates may cause a spike and crash in blood sugar. Staying in a sedentary position for hours after waking can keep metabolism sluggish. Replacing these with lighter, more balanced habits encourages steady energy.

Creating a Repeatable Routine

The benefits of morning rituals compound over time. The more consistent the routine, the easier it becomes for the body to adapt to higher energy levels and stable metabolism. Even small actions, like drinking water immediately upon waking or doing a five-minute stretch, can make a difference when repeated daily.

By focusing on gentle, sustainable practices rather than extremes, mornings can become a powerful ally in both liver health and overall energy management.

Chapter 6: Liver and Digestive Health: Fixing Common Issues

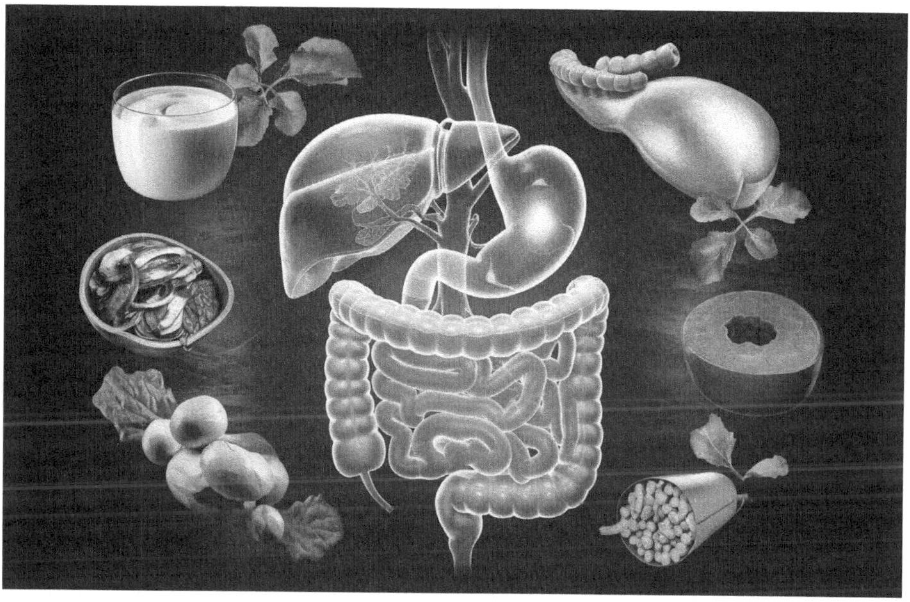

The liver and digestive system share an intimate relationship through the portal vein, which transports nutrients, metabolites, and other substances directly from the intestines to the liver. This connection, often referred to as the gut–liver axis, means that changes in gut health can have a direct impact on liver function.

1. The Gut–Liver Axis and Microbiome Balance

When the gut is balanced and healthy, the liver receives a steady flow of beneficial nutrients and minimal harmful compounds. When the gut microbiome is disturbed, harmful bacterial byproducts, inflammatory molecules, and toxins can enter the bloodstream and reach the liver, creating additional strain.

How an Imbalanced Microbiome Affects the Liver

An overgrowth of harmful bacteria, or a significant loss of beneficial species, can result in increased intestinal permeability. This condition, sometimes called "leaky gut," allows unwanted substances to pass into the bloodstream. The liver then has to work harder to filter and neutralize these compounds. Over time, this additional workload can contribute to inflammation, fat accumulation, and reduced detoxification efficiency.

Signs of Gut–Liver Imbalance

While every person's symptoms may differ, common indicators that the gut–liver axis is under stress include:

- Persistent bloating or gas
- Irregular bowel movements
- Food intolerances that develop suddenly
- Fatigue or brain fog that worsens after eating
- Skin conditions such as acne or rashes

Restoring Microbiome Balance

Improving gut health is one of the most effective ways to support the liver. This can involve:

- Increasing dietary fiber from vegetables, fruits, legumes, and whole grains to feed beneficial bacteria
- Including fermented foods like yogurt, kefir, sauerkraut, and kimchi to replenish healthy strains
- Avoiding unnecessary antibiotics and processed foods that can disrupt the microbiome
- Managing stress, as high stress levels can alter gut bacteria composition

The Role of Digestive Enzymes and Bile

The liver produces bile, which helps break down fats and assists in nutrient absorption. A healthy gut microbiome supports bile metabolism, while bile in turn influences the types of bacteria that thrive in the intestines. Disruption in either direction can set off a cycle that affects both digestion and liver function.

2. Best and Worst Foods for Digestive and Liver Health

A diet that supports both organs focuses on reducing inflammation, feeding beneficial bacteria, and providing the nutrients the liver needs to process toxins and regenerate cells. While individual needs vary, certain foods consistently appear in research for their protective effects.

- **Leafy greens and cruciferous vegetables** like spinach, kale, broccoli, and Brussels sprouts supply antioxidants and compounds that promote detoxification.
- **Berries** such as blueberries, strawberries, and blackberries are rich in polyphenols, which protect liver cells and support microbiome diversity.
- **Fatty fish** including salmon, sardines, and mackerel provide omega-3 fatty acids that lower inflammation and improve fat metabolism.
- **Legumes** like lentils, chickpeas, and black beans supply fiber and plant-based protein to support stable blood sugar and healthy gut bacteria.

- **Whole grains** such as quinoa, oats, and brown rice offer slow-releasing carbohydrates and additional fiber for digestive health.
- **Fermented foods** like sauerkraut, kimchi, kefir, and miso deliver live cultures that benefit the microbiome.

Foods to Limit or Avoid

Some foods increase inflammation, disrupt gut bacteria, and place a heavier burden on the liver. Regular consumption of these can make recovery more difficult.

- **Sugary drinks and refined sugar** feed harmful gut bacteria and contribute to fat accumulation in the liver.
- **Highly processed foods** with preservatives, artificial colors, and additives strain detox pathways.
- **Refined grains** like white bread and pasta can cause blood sugar spikes, increasing fat storage in the liver.
- **Processed meats** such as bacon, hot dogs, and deli meats often contain harmful compounds that stress liver function.
- **Fried foods** cooked in refined oils can introduce harmful oxidation products into the body.

The Importance of Cooking Methods

Even healthy foods can lose their benefits if prepared in ways that damage nutrients or introduce harmful compounds. Grilling, roasting, steaming, and light sautéing help preserve vitamins and antioxidants. Deep frying, especially in reused oils, can create inflammatory compounds that are harmful to both the liver and gut.

The Role of Variety in Gut and Liver Health

Eating a wide variety of plant-based foods is one of the best ways to maintain a healthy microbiome. Each type of plant contains different fibers and phytonutrients, which feed different bacterial strains. A diverse microbiome is better equipped to protect the gut barrier and support liver function.

People often fall into the habit of eating the same vegetables and fruits repeatedly. Rotating choices each week increases nutrient diversity and encourages a broader range of beneficial microbes to flourish.

Adjusting the Diet for Individual Needs

While general principles apply to most people, digestive and liver health can benefit from personal adjustments. Someone with frequent bloating may need to temporarily limit certain fermentable carbohydrates, while another person might require more emphasis on probiotic foods to rebuild microbiome diversity. Listening to the body's responses and making gradual changes can lead to lasting improvements.

Balancing Indulgences with Liver-Friendly Choices

It is not realistic for most people to eliminate every less-than-ideal food forever. Occasional indulgences are easier for the liver and digestive system to handle when the overall diet is nutrient-rich and supportive. Planning the majority of meals around liver-friendly and gut-friendly foods makes it possible to enjoy treats in moderation without derailing progress.

3. Probiotics, Prebiotics, and Digestive Enzymes for Healing

Probiotics are live microorganisms that help maintain a healthy balance of gut bacteria. When this balance is disrupted, harmful bacteria can flourish, leading to inflammation that affects both the digestive tract and the liver. By replenishing beneficial strains, probiotics help restore harmony in the gut–liver axis, reducing the amount of harmful byproducts that reach the liver through the portal vein.

Different probiotic strains have different benefits. For example, ***Lactobacillus plantarum*** may help improve digestion and reduce bloating, while ***Bifidobacterium longum*** can reduce inflammation and improve gut barrier integrity. Incorporating a variety of strains increases the likelihood of targeting multiple aspects of gut and liver health.

Food Sources of Probiotics

- Yogurt with live and active cultures
- Kefir, a fermented milk drink rich in diverse strains
- Sauerkraut and kimchi, which also provide beneficial enzymes
- Miso and tempeh, offering probiotic benefits along with plant-based protein
- Fermented vegetables beyond cabbage, such as carrots and beets

Not everyone tolerates all probiotic-rich foods equally, so introducing them gradually helps the digestive system adapt.

Prebiotics: Feeding the Beneficial Bacteria

Prebiotics are non-digestible fibers that serve as food for probiotics. Without adequate prebiotics, probiotic bacteria cannot thrive. These fibers pass through the upper digestive tract and are fermented by beneficial microbes in the colon, producing short-chain fatty acids that help reduce inflammation and support liver function.

Prebiotic-rich foods include garlic, onions, leeks, asparagus, bananas, artichokes, and certain whole grains like barley and oats.

Digestive Enzymes for Nutrient Absorption

Digestive enzymes help break down proteins, fats, and carbohydrates into smaller molecules that can be absorbed efficiently. When enzyme production is insufficient, food can pass into the lower digestive tract partially undigested, leading to bloating, nutrient deficiencies, and additional stress on the liver.

The body produces its own enzymes, but supplementation can be helpful in certain cases, such as after gallbladder removal or in individuals with pancreatic insufficiency.

When to Consider Supplementation

Probiotic and prebiotic supplements can be useful when dietary intake is insufficient or targeted strains are needed for a specific condition. Digestive enzyme supplements are often taken before meals to support breakdown and absorption, especially in people experiencing consistent bloating or nutrient malabsorption.

Combining Probiotics, Prebiotics, and Enzymes for Synergy

A well-rounded approach often includes all three elements: probiotics to repopulate the gut with beneficial bacteria, prebiotics to feed those bacteria, and enzymes to ensure nutrients are absorbed effectively. Together, they help reduce digestive stress, lower inflammation, and support the liver's overall workload.

4. Reducing Abdominal Bloating Naturally

Abdominal bloating can result from multiple factors, including excess gas production, water retention, poor digestion, and inflammation. For some, it may be a sign of food intolerances or imbalances in gut bacteria. The key to lasting relief is identifying and addressing the underlying cause rather than simply masking the symptom.

Dietary Adjustments to Ease Bloating

Some foods are more likely to produce gas and discomfort, especially when the gut is already sensitive. Reducing or avoiding these for a period can help pinpoint triggers.

- Carbonated drinks can introduce excess air into the digestive tract.
- Certain beans and lentils may cause gas in those with low tolerance.
- Cruciferous vegetables like broccoli and cabbage can lead to discomfort if not cooked well or introduced gradually.
- Foods high in artificial sweeteners such as sorbitol and xylitol can ferment in the gut, causing gas and bloating.

Cooking vegetables thoroughly, soaking legumes before cooking, and gradually increasing fiber intake can make digestion easier.

Mindful Eating Practices

Eating too quickly, talking while eating, or swallowing large bites of food can introduce excess air into the digestive system. This air can accumulate and cause bloating. Taking the time to chew food thoroughly allows digestive enzymes in saliva to begin breaking it down before it reaches the stomach.

It is also helpful to avoid lying down immediately after eating, as this can slow digestion and contribute to discomfort.

Hydration and Timing

Adequate water intake supports smooth digestion and helps prevent constipation, which can contribute to bloating. Drinking small amounts of water throughout the day, rather than large volumes during meals, may improve digestive comfort for some people.

Addressing Food Intolerances

Lactose, gluten, and certain high-FODMAP foods are common culprits behind persistent bloating. An elimination trial, guided by a healthcare provider or nutritionist, can help identify whether any of these are contributing factors.

The Role of Probiotics and Enzymes in Reducing Bloating

As discussed earlier, probiotics can improve the balance of gut bacteria, reducing the production of excess gas. Digestive enzymes can assist in breaking down complex foods more completely, preventing undigested particles from fermenting in the intestines.

Movement and Physical Activity

Light activity after meals, such as walking, can stimulate digestion and prevent food from lingering too long in the digestive tract. Certain yoga poses, such as gentle twists, can also help release trapped gas and ease discomfort.

Stress and Bloating

Stress can slow digestion and alter the gut microbiome, increasing the likelihood of bloating. Incorporating stress-reducing practices like deep breathing, stretching, or brief meditation sessions throughout the day can improve both digestion and liver health.

5. Linking Gut Health to Brain Fog and Mood

The gut and liver work closely together to regulate many aspects of physical health, but their influence extends into brain function and mood regulation as well. This connection is mediated by the gut–brain axis, a communication network involving the nervous system, immune system, and hormones. When gut health declines, the ripple effect can impact mental clarity and emotional stability.

The liver is central to this process because it filters and processes substances absorbed from the gut. If the gut allows excess toxins or inflammatory compounds into circulation, the liver must work harder to neutralize them. When this system is overloaded, some of these substances can reach the brain, affecting neurotransmitter balance and leading to symptoms such as brain fog or mood swings.

Brain Fog and Gut Health

Brain fog refers to a state of mental fatigue or reduced cognitive clarity. People often describe it as difficulty concentrating, slow thinking, or feeling detached. A disrupted gut microbiome can produce compounds like lipopolysaccharides, which can cross into the bloodstream when the gut lining becomes too permeable. These compounds may trigger systemic inflammation and impair brain function.

When the liver is already stressed, it may not be able to filter these inflammatory molecules efficiently, allowing them to impact brain cells and disrupt the production of chemicals involved in memory and focus.

Mood Regulation and the Microbiome

Gut bacteria play a role in producing and regulating neurotransmitters such as serotonin, dopamine, and gamma-aminobutyric acid (GABA). Around 90 percent of serotonin is produced in the gut, and disturbances in the microbiome can alter its availability. This is one reason digestive health can have such a strong influence on mood.

Chronic liver stress can add to the problem by interfering with hormone metabolism and increasing inflammatory signals. Over time, this may contribute to symptoms of anxiety, low mood, and irritability.

Identifying the Signs of Gut–Brain Imbalance

While brain fog and mood changes can result from many causes, signs that they may be linked to gut and liver health include:

- Increased mental fatigue after meals, especially high-fat or high-sugar foods
- Mood fluctuations that occur alongside digestive discomfort
- Greater difficulty concentrating during periods of bloating or abdominal discomfort
- Changes in mental clarity during times of poor diet or disrupted sleep

Approaches to Improve Mental Clarity and Mood Through Gut Support

While improvement requires a holistic approach, certain strategies can begin to restore balance:

- Eating a wide variety of fiber-rich plant foods to support a healthy microbiome
- Including probiotic-rich foods or supplements to help restore beneficial bacteria
- Avoiding highly processed foods and added sugars that feed harmful bacteria
- Staying hydrated to assist digestion and nutrient transport
- Incorporating stress-management techniques, as stress impacts both gut and brain health

6. Functional Medicine Tools for Gut–Liver Repair

Functional medicine looks at the body as an interconnected system rather than isolated organs. The gut and liver are a prime example of this approach. Improving one often requires attention to the other. This perspective uses targeted testing, dietary interventions, and lifestyle adjustments to identify and correct the underlying imbalances driving symptoms.

Personalized Assessment

The first step in functional medicine is thorough evaluation. This often includes:

- Advanced stool analysis to assess gut bacteria balance, digestive capacity, and inflammation markers
- Food sensitivity testing to identify dietary triggers
- Liver function panels to measure enzymes, bilirubin, and protein production
- Micronutrient testing to detect deficiencies that affect repair and regeneration

This data allows for a plan tailored to the individual's specific needs rather than a one-size-fits-all approach.

Targeted Nutrition Plans

Functional medicine emphasizes nutrient-dense, anti-inflammatory foods. These plans often combine gut-supportive and liver-healing strategies. For example, cruciferous vegetables provide compounds that aid both liver detoxification and gut microbiome diversity. High-fiber foods not only promote bowel regularity but also help the liver by reducing the reabsorption of toxins through the digestive tract.

Probiotics, Prebiotics, and Digestive Enzymes in Practice

While these elements have been discussed individually, functional medicine combines them strategically. Probiotics may be chosen based on specific deficiencies found in testing. Prebiotics are introduced gradually to avoid discomfort while still feeding beneficial bacteria. Digestive enzymes are added if testing suggests poor breakdown of proteins, fats, or carbohydrates.

Detoxification Support

Rather than aggressive cleanses, functional medicine focuses on sustainable detoxification support. This may include:

- Hydration protocols to assist kidney and bowel elimination
- Specific herbs like milk thistle or dandelion root to support bile flow and antioxidant defenses

- Adequate protein intake to ensure the liver has the amino acids needed for detoxification enzymes
- Encouraging sweating through light exercise or sauna use to assist toxin elimination through the skin

Restoring Gut Barrier Function

A healthy gut barrier prevents harmful substances from reaching the liver. Functional medicine may recommend nutrients like glutamine, zinc, and omega-3 fatty acids to repair and maintain this barrier. Collagen-rich foods or supplements can also help strengthen the gut lining.

Lifestyle Interventions

Functional medicine acknowledges that lifestyle factors heavily influence gut–liver health. Improving sleep quality allows the liver to perform overnight detoxification, while stress reduction techniques reduce cortisol-driven inflammation. Regular movement enhances circulation between the gut and liver, aiding nutrient delivery and toxin removal.

Long-Term Maintenance

Gut and liver repair is not a quick process. Functional medicine practitioners often emphasize gradual, sustainable changes that can be maintained for life. This might involve rotating probiotic strains, continuing a diverse diet, and maintaining a consistent exercise routine. The goal is not just symptom relief but creating a stable foundation for ongoing health.

Chapter 7: Inflammation and Liver Health: Preventing Long-Term Damage

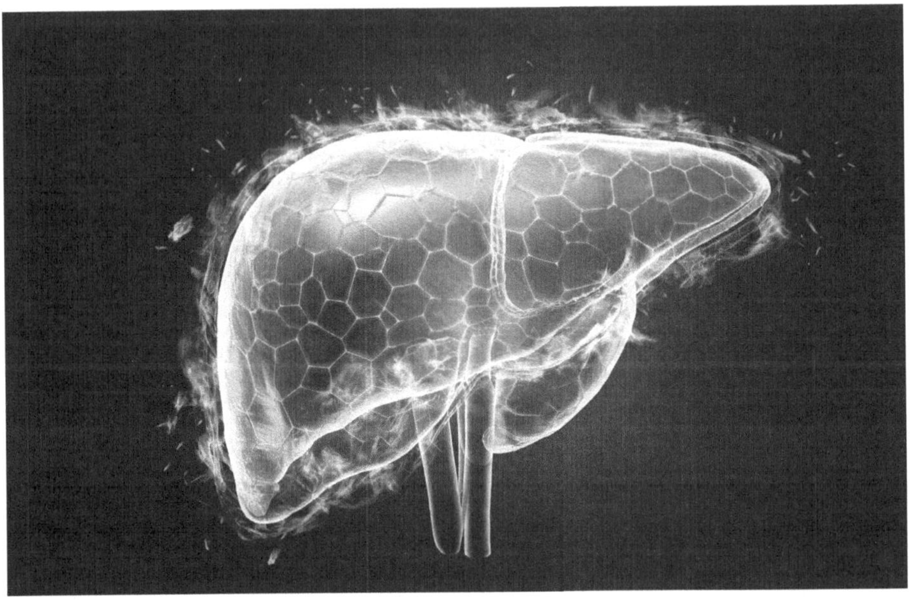

Inflammation is the body's way of responding to injury or infection. In the short term, it helps repair tissue and fight harmful invaders. However, when inflammation becomes chronic, it stops being protective and starts causing harm. In the liver, this process can quietly progress for years, leading to lasting structural changes and loss of function.

1. How Chronic Inflammation Damages the Liver

The liver is exposed to a constant stream of compounds from the digestive tract. If these include harmful substances, toxins, or excess inflammatory molecules, liver cells (hepatocytes) activate immune responses to neutralize the threat. When these responses are prolonged, healthy cells can be caught in the crossfire, leading to scarring and reduced function.

The Link Between Inflammation and Fatty Liver

Fatty liver disease, both alcoholic and non-alcoholic, often begins with fat accumulation. Once fat is stored in the liver cells, it can trigger immune activity. Fat cells release inflammatory cytokines, which activate the body's immune defense. Over time, this low-grade inflammation becomes constant, damaging liver tissue and encouraging the progression from simple steatosis to more advanced conditions such as non-alcoholic steatohepatitis (NASH).

When inflammation persists, fibrotic tissue begins to replace healthy liver cells. This scarring restricts blood flow within the liver, further reducing its ability to perform essential tasks like detoxification, bile production, and nutrient processing.

How Chronic Inflammation Creates a Cycle of Damage

Once inflammation starts harming the liver, it often creates a cycle that feeds itself:

1. Fat or toxins irritate liver cells.
2. The immune system responds, producing inflammatory molecules.
3. Healthy liver tissue is damaged in the process.
4. Scar tissue develops, which reduces liver efficiency.
5. Poor function leads to further buildup of fat and toxins.
6. The cycle repeats, causing progressive damage over time.

Sources of Ongoing Inflammation

Some factors can keep inflammation active in the liver for years if not addressed:

- Diets high in processed sugars and refined carbohydrates
- Excessive alcohol consumption
- Chronic viral infections such as hepatitis B or C
- Environmental toxins from food packaging, pesticides, and pollution
- Long-term use of certain medications
- Poor gut health leading to increased intestinal permeability and toxin leakage into the bloodstream

The Role of Oxidative Stress

Oxidative stress occurs when there is an imbalance between free radicals and antioxidants in the body. Chronic inflammation often increases free radical production in the liver. Over time, these unstable molecules damage cell membranes, proteins, and DNA, further weakening liver function. Without enough antioxidant defenses, the damage accumulates.

Why Early Intervention Matters

Chronic inflammation can be silent. Many people do not feel any symptoms until significant damage has already occurred. This is why addressing inflammation early through diet, lifestyle, and targeted nutrients is essential for preventing irreversible conditions like cirrhosis or liver cancer.

2. Anti-Inflammatory Foods that Support Liver Function

The liver is directly influenced by what passes through the digestive system. Foods can either fuel inflammation or help control it. A diet focused on anti-inflammatory ingredients not only protects the liver but also supports its regeneration and detoxification abilities.

Incorporating these foods into daily meals helps reduce oxidative stress, modulate the immune response, and maintain healthy fat levels in liver cells.

Key Anti-Inflammatory Foods for Liver Health

- **Leafy greens** such as spinach, kale, and arugula contain chlorophyll and antioxidants that help neutralize toxins and protect cells.
- **Berries** including blueberries, blackberries, and strawberries are rich in polyphenols and vitamin C, which reduce oxidative stress and support collagen production in liver tissue.
- **Fatty fish** like salmon, sardines, and mackerel provide omega-3 fatty acids that reduce inflammation and improve fat metabolism.
- **Turmeric** contains curcumin, a compound that modulates inflammatory pathways and supports bile production.
- **Garlic and onions** are rich in sulfur compounds that help activate detoxification enzymes and lower inflammation.
- **Olive oil** offers monounsaturated fats and antioxidants that protect against oxidative damage and improve lipid profiles.
- **Nuts and seeds** such as walnuts, flaxseeds, and chia seeds provide omega-3s and fiber that support metabolic health.
- **Green tea** contains catechins, powerful antioxidants that have been studied for their role in reducing fat accumulation and inflammation in the liver.

The Role of Fiber

A diet high in fiber helps reduce inflammation by promoting healthy gut bacteria and preventing constipation. This limits the reabsorption of toxins into the bloodstream, reducing the load on the liver. Soluble fiber, found in oats, legumes, and certain fruits, is particularly beneficial for improving cholesterol levels and supporting stable blood sugar.

Cooking Methods That Preserve Benefits

The way food is prepared can influence its anti-inflammatory potential. Steaming, light sautéing, and roasting at moderate temperatures help preserve antioxidants and beneficial fats. Overcooking vegetables or frying foods in refined oils can destroy these protective compounds and create harmful oxidation products.

Balancing Macronutrients for Liver Healing

While the focus is often on specific anti-inflammatory foods, the overall balance of carbohydrates, proteins, and fats matters as well.

- **Complex carbohydrates** from whole grains and vegetables provide steady energy without spiking blood sugar.
- **High-quality proteins** from fish, poultry, legumes, and eggs provide amino acids needed for repair.
- **Healthy fats** from nuts, seeds, avocados, and olive oil help control inflammation and support hormone balance.

Incorporating Anti-Inflammatory Herbs and Spices

Many herbs and spices contain concentrated anti-inflammatory compounds. Cinnamon, rosemary, ginger, and oregano can easily be added to meals to increase their health benefits. These additions not only support liver function but also improve digestion and flavor, making it easier to maintain a healing diet long term.

Making Anti-Inflammatory Eating a Daily Habit

Small, consistent changes often have the greatest impact. This can mean replacing refined cooking oils with extra virgin olive oil, adding berries to breakfast, or including a side of steamed greens with lunch or dinner. Over time, these simple choices help lower inflammation and create a more supportive environment for liver health.

3. Omega-3s, Antioxidants, and Polyphenols for Repair

Fatty liver disease, whether caused by poor diet, metabolic imbalance, or other factors, involves two main issues: fat accumulation and chronic inflammation. Omega-3 fatty acids, antioxidants, and polyphenols directly address these challenges. Omega-3s help reduce liver fat and inflammation. Antioxidants protect cells from oxidative stress, which is a major driver of liver damage. Polyphenols modulate inflammatory pathways and support liver regeneration. Together, they create a powerful nutritional foundation for healing.

Omega-3 Fatty Acids

Omega-3s are essential fats the body cannot produce on its own. They are known for their anti-inflammatory effects, but their benefits for liver health go even further.

They improve triglyceride levels, help balance cholesterol ratios, and may prevent fat from accumulating in the liver. Research shows that people with non-alcoholic fatty liver disease (NAFLD) who increase omega-3 intake often see reductions in liver fat and improved enzyme levels.

Sources of Omega-3s include:

- Fatty fish such as salmon, sardines, mackerel, and trout
- Plant-based sources like chia seeds, flaxseeds, hemp seeds, and walnuts

- Algal oil supplements for those who do not consume fish

Including omega-3-rich foods at least twice a week or supplementing under guidance can be a practical way to support liver repair.

Antioxidants and Liver Protection

The liver is constantly exposed to oxidative stress as it processes toxins, medications, and metabolic byproducts. Antioxidants neutralize free radicals, preventing them from damaging liver cells. This protection is critical for people working to reverse fatty liver and reduce inflammation.

Vitamin C supports collagen production in the liver's connective tissue and enhances immune function. Vitamin E is fat-soluble, making it particularly effective at protecting cell membranes in fatty liver conditions. Selenium helps maintain the liver's antioxidant defenses by supporting glutathione production, one of the body's most important natural antioxidants.

Foods rich in antioxidants include:

- Citrus fruits, strawberries, and kiwifruit for vitamin C
- Almonds, sunflower seeds, and avocado for vitamin E
- Brazil nuts and seafood for selenium

Polyphenols for Regeneration

Polyphenols are plant compounds that influence multiple pathways in the body. They help lower inflammation, improve blood sugar control, and protect blood vessels. In the context of liver health, polyphenols have been shown to improve fat metabolism and reduce fibrosis risk.

Green tea is a notable source, containing catechins that reduce fat buildup and improve enzyme profiles. Berries offer anthocyanins, which lower oxidative stress and inflammation. Dark chocolate (with high cocoa content) contains flavonoids that may support vascular health and reduce liver stress when consumed in moderation.

Integrating These Nutrients Into Daily Eating

A meal plan for liver regeneration can include grilled salmon with steamed vegetables, a side salad with walnuts, and a cup of green tea. Breakfast might feature oatmeal with blueberries, ground flaxseed, and a sprinkling of cinnamon for additional antioxidant support. Snacks can include a small handful of almonds or a square of dark chocolate alongside herbal tea.

By making these foods a consistent part of the diet, the liver's repair processes are supported naturally without relying solely on supplements.

4. Lifestyle Habits to Lower Inflammation

Diet is only part of the anti-inflammatory approach. Everyday lifestyle choices have a direct effect on liver health and the body's ability to reverse fatty liver. Regular movement, restorative sleep, and stress management all influence inflammation levels. Ignoring these areas can slow progress, even if the diet is optimal.

Physical Activity to Reduce Liver Inflammation

Exercise improves insulin sensitivity, promotes fat burning, and reduces circulating inflammatory markers. For liver health, the goal is not extreme training but consistent movement.

Moderate-intensity aerobic exercise, such as brisk walking, swimming, or cycling, has been shown to lower liver fat levels in people with NAFLD. Strength training helps maintain lean muscle mass, which boosts metabolism and makes blood sugar easier to regulate.

A realistic approach might include 30 minutes of walking five days per week, paired with two sessions of resistance exercises. The focus should be on building a routine that is sustainable, not overwhelming.

Sleep as a Foundation for Recovery

Poor sleep increases cortisol and inflammatory markers while disrupting blood sugar balance. The liver does much of its detoxification and repair work during deep sleep, so inadequate rest can hinder regeneration.

Creating a consistent sleep schedule, keeping the bedroom cool and dark, and avoiding heavy meals or caffeine close to bedtime can make a significant difference. For some, gentle stretching or breathing exercises before bed help the body wind down, making sleep deeper and more restorative.

Stress Reduction and Cortisol Balance

Chronic stress is a hidden driver of inflammation. High cortisol levels over time can encourage fat storage in the liver and abdomen, weaken immunity, and slow healing. Stress management does not require elaborate programs; simple, consistent practices are often enough.

Breathing exercises, meditation, light yoga, or even short nature walks can all help reset the nervous system. Taking breaks during the day, staying connected with supportive people, and engaging in hobbies that bring enjoyment also help lower stress hormones naturally.

Limiting Toxin Exposure in Daily Life

Environmental toxins, including pesticides, chemical cleaners, and certain plastics, add to the liver's workload. Choosing organic produce when possible, switching to natural cleaning products, and avoiding unnecessary medications all help reduce the toxic burden. Using glass or stainless steel instead of plastic containers can also lower exposure to harmful compounds.

Hydration for Inflammation Control

Water aids circulation, nutrient delivery, and waste elimination. Staying hydrated supports the kidneys in removing inflammatory byproducts and helps maintain healthy bile flow for digestion. For most adults, drinking water regularly throughout the day, rather than in large amounts at once, is most effective.

Consistency Over Perfection

Lowering inflammation is not about doing everything perfectly every single day. It is about making consistent, sustainable choices that create a healthier baseline over time. Small daily actions, such as adding an extra serving of vegetables, taking a short walk, or replacing one processed snack with a nutrient-rich option, can build momentum toward lasting liver health and reduced inflammation.

5. Tracking Inflammation Markers Over Time

In fatty liver disease and other liver-related conditions, inflammation is often the silent driver of damage. You may feel fine, yet inside, inflammatory activity can be steadily harming cells and encouraging scar tissue formation. Tracking inflammation markers over time allows you to see whether your diet, supplements, and lifestyle strategies are reducing this underlying threat.

For many people, this tracking also reinforces motivation. Seeing certain markers improve alongside better digestion, energy, and mental clarity can be a powerful confirmation that the body is moving toward healing.

Commonly Used Inflammation Markers

There are several blood tests that can provide insight into systemic inflammation and how it might be affecting the liver.

- **C-reactive protein (CRP)** is one of the most common tests. High-sensitivity CRP (hs-CRP) can detect low-grade inflammation, which is important in metabolic conditions like fatty liver disease.
- **Erythrocyte sedimentation rate (ESR)** measures how quickly red blood cells settle in a tube of blood. A faster rate can signal inflammation.
- **Ferritin** is often thought of as an iron storage marker, but it can also rise in response to inflammation.
- **Liver enzyme patterns** such as persistent ALT or AST elevation can indicate liver inflammation when paired with other clinical findings.

Establishing a Baseline

Before making changes to reverse fatty liver or reduce liver inflammation, it is important to have a starting point. This baseline helps measure progress accurately. Without a clear baseline, improvements or setbacks may go unnoticed.

A good starting assessment might include hs-CRP, liver enzymes, fasting blood sugar, fasting insulin, and a lipid profile. For some, additional testing like ferritin or fasting homocysteine may be recommended, particularly if there are risk factors for cardiovascular or metabolic disease.

Frequency of Testing

The ideal frequency for retesting depends on the severity of the condition and the treatment plan. For those making significant dietary or lifestyle changes, repeating tests every three to six months is common. This timeframe is long enough to see real changes but short enough to make adjustments if progress is slow.

Interpreting Trends, Not Just Numbers

It is important to focus on the direction of change rather than one isolated result. A small, steady decline in hs-CRP over several tests is more meaningful than a single sharp drop that is not sustained. Trends help determine whether your anti-inflammatory diet, supplements, or metabolic reset program is truly working.

Sometimes you may see improvements in symptoms before blood markers change, while in other cases, the blood markers improve first. Both situations are valuable clues that the body is responding.

Working with a Healthcare Professional

A qualified healthcare provider can help interpret results in context. For example, a slightly elevated ferritin might not be concerning if iron status is high but stable. However, the same ferritin level paired with high CRP could point toward an inflammatory process that needs further attention. Professional guidance ensures you are responding to the right signals without overreacting to normal variations.

6. Inflammation and Insulin Resistance Connection

Chronic inflammation affects how cells respond to insulin, the hormone responsible for moving glucose out of the bloodstream and into cells for energy. Inflammatory molecules can interfere with insulin signaling pathways, making it harder for glucose to enter cells. The pancreas compensates by producing more insulin, which leads to higher circulating insulin levels.

This insulin resistance creates a vicious cycle in fatty liver disease. Elevated insulin promotes more fat storage in the liver, and the excess fat itself triggers further inflammation.

Why This Connection Matters for Liver Health

In people with non-alcoholic fatty liver disease, insulin resistance is a key driver of progression from simple fat accumulation to more advanced stages involving inflammation and fibrosis. Addressing both inflammation and insulin resistance is essential for reversing fatty liver and preventing long-term complications.

If only one is targeted, progress can be limited. For example, lowering inflammation without improving insulin sensitivity may still allow fat to accumulate in the liver. Likewise, improving insulin sensitivity without reducing inflammation leaves the liver vulnerable to ongoing cellular damage.

Dietary Approaches That Target Both

Some foods and eating patterns reduce inflammation while also improving insulin function.

- A diet rich in colorful vegetables and low-sugar fruits provides antioxidants and fiber to reduce inflammatory stress.
- Lean proteins like fish, poultry, and legumes support stable blood sugar and supply amino acids for repair.
- Healthy fats from nuts, seeds, olive oil, and fatty fish reduce inflammatory markers and improve insulin sensitivity.
- Minimizing refined carbohydrates and added sugars helps prevent insulin spikes that feed the fatty liver cycle.

The Role of Physical Activity

Exercise is one of the most powerful tools for addressing this dual problem. It improves insulin sensitivity immediately after activity and over the long term, especially when done consistently. Moderate-intensity aerobic exercise, combined with strength training, can lower inflammatory markers while also helping the liver metabolize stored fat.

Weight Management and Visceral Fat

Excess abdominal fat is strongly linked to both insulin resistance and inflammation. Even a modest weight loss of 5 to 10 percent can improve liver enzyme levels, lower CRP, and enhance insulin function. This is not about extreme dieting but about sustainable changes that create steady progress toward a healthier weight.

Stress, Sleep, and Hormonal Balance

Chronic stress and poor sleep raise cortisol levels, which in turn worsen both inflammation and insulin resistance. Establishing a consistent sleep routine and incorporating stress-reducing activities can help break this cycle. Simple practices like walking outdoors, deep breathing, or gentle stretching before bed can make a measurable difference.

Breaking the Cycle for Long-Term Healing

Reducing liver inflammation and reversing insulin resistance require an integrated approach that combines diet, physical activity, weight management, and lifestyle adjustments. The improvements may be gradual, but over time they reinforce one another, moving the body toward better liver health, balanced blood sugar, and a lower risk of metabolic complications.

Part 3

The Natural Liver Healing Method

Chapter 8: Debunking Liver Detox Myths: What Really Works?

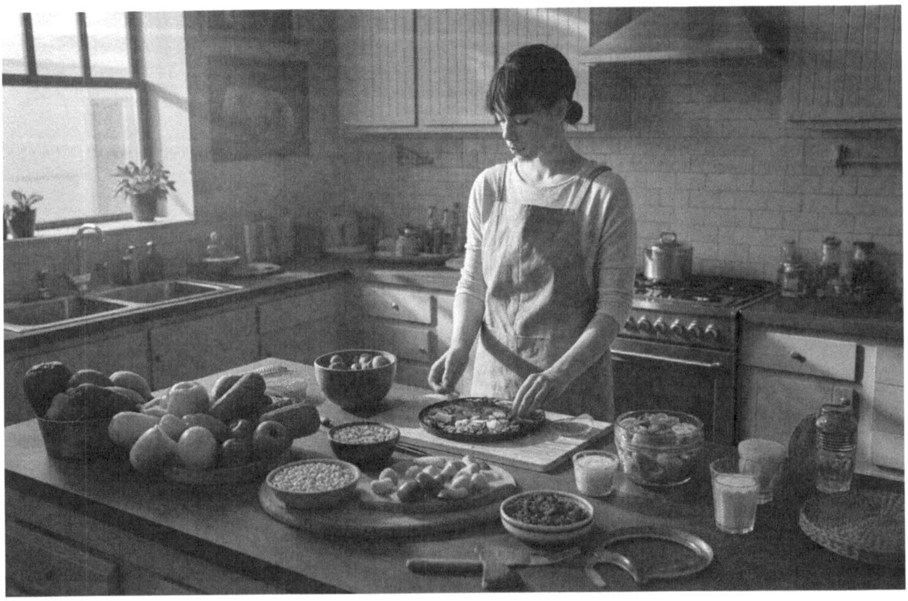

The liver is naturally equipped to detox your body every single day. It processes nutrients from food, breaks down toxins, and neutralizes harmful chemicals from the environment. This is done through two main phases of detoxification, supported by a complex network of enzymes, antioxidants, and other compounds.

Phase one changes toxins into intermediate forms, often making them more chemically active. Phase two binds these intermediates to other molecules, making them water-soluble so they can be removed through urine or bile. This is an ongoing process, not something the liver turns on only when you decide to do a cleanse.

1. Does the Liver Actually Need Detoxing? Science Explains

The popularity of "liver detox" products and extreme cleanses comes from the idea that the liver is like a dirty filter that needs to be flushed clean. In reality, the liver does not store toxins in the way a filter stores debris. Instead, it transforms them so they can be excreted. The problem arises when the liver is overburdened by excessive exposure to harmful substances or lacks the nutrients needed for efficient detoxification.

When the Liver's Detox Capacity Is Compromised

Although the liver does not technically need "detoxing" in the sense of a complete reset, its natural detox processes can slow down or become less effective. This happens in cases of fatty liver disease, high toxin exposure, nutrient deficiencies, and chronic inflammation.

If these conditions persist, the body may struggle to clear waste efficiently, leading to symptoms such as fatigue, brain fog, skin issues, and digestive discomfort. In these situations, supporting the liver with proper nutrition, hydration, and lifestyle changes can help restore its optimal function.

Why Quick-Fix Cleanses Fall Short

Many marketed cleanses involve fasting, consuming only juices, or using harsh herbal laxatives. While they may cause temporary weight loss or make you feel lighter, they often fail to provide the protein, antioxidants, and essential nutrients the liver needs to function well. In some cases, these extreme cleanses can even stress the liver further, especially in people with existing conditions.

The Science-Based Approach to Liver Support

Instead of trying to "detox" the liver in a dramatic way, the goal should be to give it the right conditions to do its job efficiently. This means:

- Providing the nutrients it needs for both detox phases
- Reducing unnecessary toxin exposure
- Supporting healthy digestion so waste products leave the body quickly
- Maintaining steady blood sugar to prevent fat buildup in liver cells

2. Safe and Effective Detox Strategies Backed by Research

The liver's detoxification system depends on a constant supply of nutrients. Phase one requires B vitamins, certain amino acids, and antioxidants like vitamin C. Phase two relies on sulfur-containing compounds from foods like garlic, onions, broccoli, and kale. Without these nutrients, detox pathways can become imbalanced.

Ensuring your diet contains a variety of colorful vegetables, high-quality proteins, and healthy fats gives the liver the tools it needs to perform continuous detoxification.

Hydration and Waste Removal

Water is essential for flushing out water-soluble toxins. When hydration is poor, the kidneys cannot efficiently eliminate waste, and the colon may also slow down. This can lead to toxins being reabsorbed into the bloodstream, increasing the liver's workload. Drinking water consistently throughout the day supports both kidney and liver function.

Fiber for Binding and Elimination

Fiber binds to certain toxins and waste products in the digestive tract, preventing them from being reabsorbed. It also promotes regular bowel movements, which is critical for detoxification. Foods like flaxseed, chia seeds, oats, beans, and leafy greens are excellent fiber sources. A liver-friendly diet plan should include both soluble and insoluble fiber for maximum benefit.

Supporting Bile Flow

Bile is one of the main routes for removing fat-soluble toxins. Foods that stimulate bile production, such as beets, artichokes, dandelion greens, and lemon water, can improve detox efficiency. Regular bile flow also supports digestion and nutrient absorption, which indirectly benefits liver regeneration.

Gentle Herbal Support

Some herbs have been shown to support liver health without the harsh side effects of extreme cleanses.

- **Milk thistle** may protect liver cells from toxins and support regeneration.
- **Turmeric** can reduce inflammation and improve bile flow.
- **Dandelion root** has mild diuretic properties and may aid detox pathways.

These should be used as part of a broader liver health guide rather than as the sole strategy.

Reducing the Inflammatory Load

An anti-inflammatory diet can reduce the background stress that interferes with liver function. This means focusing on whole foods, avoiding processed sugars, and balancing omega-3 to omega-6 fats. Lowering inflammation helps the liver prioritize detoxification and repair instead of dealing with constant damage.

Limiting Environmental Toxins

You cannot avoid all toxins, but you can reduce exposure to common sources.

- Choose fresh or frozen foods instead of heavily packaged items with additives.
- Use natural cleaning products to avoid harsh chemicals.
- Avoid heating food in plastic containers to reduce chemical leaching.

Small steps like these reduce the burden on detox systems over time.

Physical Activity and Circulation

Movement improves circulation, ensuring that nutrients and oxygen reach the liver while waste products are carried away efficiently. Moderate exercise also promotes sweating, which can help remove certain compounds through the skin. Walking, swimming, or yoga can all be effective for supporting detox without straining the body.

Making Detox a Daily Practice

The most effective detox plan is not a one-time event but an ongoing lifestyle. Eating nutrient-dense meals, staying hydrated, moving regularly, and limiting toxin exposure create a consistent environment for the liver to thrive. Over time, these habits help reverse fatty liver, reduce liver inflammation, and support long-term metabolic health.

3. Why "Extreme Cleanses" May Harm Liver Health

Many popular cleanses promise to flush toxins from the body within a few days, often by restricting food to juices, herbal drinks, or very low-calorie diets. While these approaches may seem appealing for quick results, they can actually slow liver regeneration and interfere with its ability to function properly. The liver needs a steady supply of protein, antioxidants, vitamins, and minerals to complete its detoxification cycles. When these are missing, detox pathways can stall, leaving partially processed toxins circulating in the body.

Impact on Blood Sugar and Energy

Most extreme cleanses provide too few calories to maintain stable blood sugar. Without complex carbohydrates and balanced protein, the liver cannot keep glycogen stores steady, which means blood sugar drops more quickly. This can lead to dizziness, irritability, fatigue, and mental fog. Over time, repeated episodes of unstable blood sugar can contribute to metabolic imbalances, which are closely linked to fatty liver disease.

Nutrient Depletion

The detoxification process in the liver's two phases requires specific nutrients such as B vitamins, amino acids, sulfur compounds, and antioxidants. Extreme cleanses often lack adequate sources of these, particularly if they eliminate whole food groups for several days or weeks. Without these essential building blocks, the body may process toxins in phase one but fail to complete phase two, which binds and removes them. This incomplete process may leave the body more vulnerable to oxidative stress and inflammation.

Stress on the Digestive System

Some cleanses involve strong laxatives or herbal combinations that stimulate bowel movements aggressively. While this may create a temporary feeling of lightness, it can also cause dehydration, electrolyte imbalance, and irritation of the digestive tract. For someone already experiencing digestive issues or reduced bile flow, this added stress can worsen symptoms rather than improve them.

Risk of Overloading the Liver

If a cleanse triggers a sudden release of stored toxins from fat tissue, the liver may be overwhelmed by the increased load. This is particularly risky for people with fatty liver disease or other existing liver conditions. Without proper nutritional and antioxidant support, the liver's natural detox systems may not keep pace with the sudden influx of compounds, potentially increasing oxidative damage.

Why the Quick-Fix Mentality is Misleading

The marketing behind extreme cleanses often implies that toxins can be eliminated all at once, as if the liver can be "reset" like a machine. In reality, detoxification is a daily process that works best when supported continuously, not forced through extreme or unsafe methods. A focus on long-term lifestyle changes is more effective for reversing fatty liver and reducing liver inflammation.

4. Gentle Detox Practices for Beginners

For those who want to improve liver health and detox the body without overwhelming it, a gentle, nutrient-supportive plan is the safest choice. Gentle detox practices help the liver work efficiently without depriving it of essential resources. They also fit more easily into daily life, making them sustainable in the long run.

Start with Hydration

Water supports kidney function and helps flush water-soluble toxins from the body. Consistent hydration also keeps bile fluid, which assists in the removal of fat-soluble toxins through digestion. Adding a slice of lemon or a splash of apple cider vinegar to water can encourage bile flow without harsh effects.

Increase Whole, Unprocessed Foods

Replacing processed snacks and sugary drinks with whole foods immediately reduces the intake of harmful additives, preservatives, and excess sugars. These changes help reduce the liver's toxin load and stabilize blood sugar. Focus on vegetables, fruits, legumes, whole grains, lean proteins, and healthy fats.

Fiber as a Gentle Detox Aid

Dietary fiber binds certain waste products in the gut and helps move them out of the body. Soluble fiber from oats, beans, and apples is especially useful for binding bile acids, while insoluble fiber from leafy greens, carrots, and whole grains supports bowel regularity. Increasing fiber gradually is important to avoid digestive discomfort.

Support Bile Flow Naturally

Bile is essential for breaking down dietary fats and carrying fat-soluble toxins out of the body. Foods that encourage bile production include beets, artichokes, bitter greens like dandelion leaves, and small amounts of healthy fats such as olive oil or avocado. A consistent intake of these foods helps maintain healthy liver and gallbladder function.

Include Gentle Herbal Support

Beginners can incorporate herbs that have a mild but supportive effect on the liver without overloading it.

- **Milk thistle** can help protect liver cells and encourage regeneration.
- **Turmeric** may reduce inflammation and support bile flow.
- **Ginger** aids digestion and has mild anti-inflammatory properties.

These herbs can be included as teas, culinary ingredients, or supplements under professional guidance.

Light Movement to Aid Circulation

Gentle physical activity improves blood flow to the liver and other organs, helping distribute nutrients and remove waste products more effectively. Walking, stretching, or yoga can all be part of a daily routine that supports detoxification.

Manage Stress for Better Detox Efficiency

Stress triggers hormonal changes that can slow digestion and alter liver metabolism. Practicing mindfulness, deep breathing, or even brief periods of quiet reflection each day can lower stress hormones and give the liver a better environment for detox and regeneration.

Sleep as a Detox Ally

The liver is highly active during deep sleep, processing toxins and performing repair work. Establishing a regular sleep schedule and creating a calm, dark sleeping environment ensures the liver has time to perform these critical functions.

Making Gentle Detox a Habit

Rather than committing to short-term, high-intensity cleanses, beginners can start by adopting one or two of these practices each week and gradually building them into daily life. Over time, the cumulative effect of consistent hydration, nutrient-rich meals, and supportive lifestyle habits will help reverse fatty liver, reduce liver inflammation, and improve overall energy and digestion.

5. Environmental and Lifestyle Detox Factors

The liver's detox workload is shaped not only by diet but also by the environment you live in and the habits you keep. Chemicals in household products, pesticides on produce, fumes from cleaning agents, and even some personal care items can add to the body's toxic burden. Each extra compound the liver must neutralize takes away energy and resources from other important tasks like regeneration and fat metabolism.

Many people underestimate how much low-level, long-term exposure can contribute to fatigue, hormonal imbalances, and the progression of fatty liver disease. Reducing these exposures is one of the most effective ways to give the liver space to heal.

Household and Personal Care Products

A large number of cleaning products, air fresheners, and scented candles contain volatile organic compounds (VOCs) that are inhaled or absorbed through the skin. These compounds travel through the bloodstream and end up in the liver for processing. Switching to fragrance-free or plant-based alternatives reduces this strain. Similarly, many cosmetics, shampoos, and lotions include parabens, phthalates, or synthetic fragrances that are best avoided when supporting liver health.

Air and Water Quality

The air inside homes and workplaces can sometimes contain more pollutants than outdoor air. Dust, mold spores, and fumes from synthetic materials accumulate in enclosed spaces. Opening windows when possible, using high-quality air filters, and keeping indoor plants can improve air quality.

Water is another important factor. Tap water may contain chlorine, fluoride, heavy metals, or traces of pesticides. Using a reliable water filter can help reduce these exposures and ensure hydration supports, rather than challenges, the detox process.

Pesticides and Food Safety

Produce grown with conventional farming methods often carries pesticide residues. While washing fruits and vegetables helps, it may not remove all residues. Choosing organic options for high-pesticide items or buying from local farms that use low-spray practices can help lower toxin intake. Storing food in glass containers instead of plastic reduces exposure to chemicals like BPA, which can leach into food.

Lifestyle Habits That Influence Detox Load

Beyond environmental exposures, certain lifestyle habits also play a role in how efficiently the liver can perform its work. Excessive alcohol use, frequent consumption of processed foods, and irregular sleep patterns all increase liver stress. Long periods of inactivity slow circulation and lymphatic flow, making it harder for the body to move toxins toward elimination.

Even small adjustments, such as replacing a daily sugary beverage with water or scheduling short activity breaks throughout the day, can significantly reduce the liver's workload.

The Role of Stress and Emotional Health

Stress does not just affect the mind; it changes the way the body processes and stores toxins. Elevated cortisol levels can alter liver metabolism, leading to more fat storage and slower detoxification. Chronic stress also affects digestion, increasing the risk of gut permeability and allowing more toxins to enter circulation. This makes stress management a critical part of any liver regeneration or detox program.

6. Long-Term Detoxification Support

Detoxification is not a short-term event. The liver works around the clock to process everything that enters the bloodstream, from nutrients to environmental chemicals. While short-term cleanses can offer a starting point, lasting results come from daily habits that consistently lighten the liver's burden and enhance its performance.

Building a Detox-Friendly Diet

A long-term liver cleanse approach centers on an anti-inflammatory diet rich in vegetables, fruits, legumes, whole grains, healthy fats, and lean proteins. This kind of eating pattern provides a steady supply of vitamins, minerals, antioxidants, and amino acids needed for both phases of detoxification.

Foods like cruciferous vegetables (broccoli, kale, Brussels sprouts) are particularly valuable for activating detox enzymes. Citrus fruits provide vitamin C, which supports antioxidant activity. Garlic and onions supply sulfur compounds essential for binding toxins in phase two of detox.

Regular Movement for Circulation and Lymph Flow

The liver depends on healthy circulation to receive nutrients and remove waste efficiently. Daily physical activity improves blood flow, stimulates lymphatic drainage, and supports healthy digestion. Walking, swimming, cycling, and stretching all encourage the body's natural detox systems to work at full capacity without overstressing the liver.

Hydration as a Non-Negotiable

Water is a simple but powerful tool for detox your body routines. It ensures waste products are carried out through the kidneys and supports healthy bile flow for fat-soluble toxin removal. For many people, aiming for steady hydration throughout the day is more effective than drinking large amounts at once. Herbal teas like dandelion root or green tea can add an extra layer of support.

Sleep and Repair Cycles

Deep sleep is when the liver performs much of its repair and regeneration work. This is also when the brain's glymphatic system clears waste from the nervous system, reducing overall inflammation. Going to bed at a consistent time and creating a dark, quiet sleeping space helps maximize these overnight detox processes.

Managing Toxin Exposure Long-Term

Once initial environmental improvements have been made, it is important to maintain them. This means continuing to choose safer cleaning products, monitoring indoor air quality, and staying mindful about food sourcing. Over time, these consistent decisions lead to a lighter toxin load and a healthier, more resilient liver.

Incorporating Gentle Herbal and Nutritional Support

Certain herbs and nutrients can be taken long-term to promote liver health without causing dependency or stress on the system. Milk thistle, turmeric, and artichoke leaf are gentle enough for extended use under professional guidance. Nutrients like magnesium, zinc, and selenium can also be beneficial, particularly if deficiencies are present.

Sustainable Habits Over Short-Term Fixes

The most effective long-term detox plan is one that becomes part of your lifestyle. This is not about perfection but about making enough consistent, supportive choices that the liver is never pushed beyond its capacity. A balanced diet, regular exercise, restful sleep, hydration, and toxin reduction together create an environment where liver regeneration is possible and sustained.

Chapter 9: Nutrition for Liver Healing

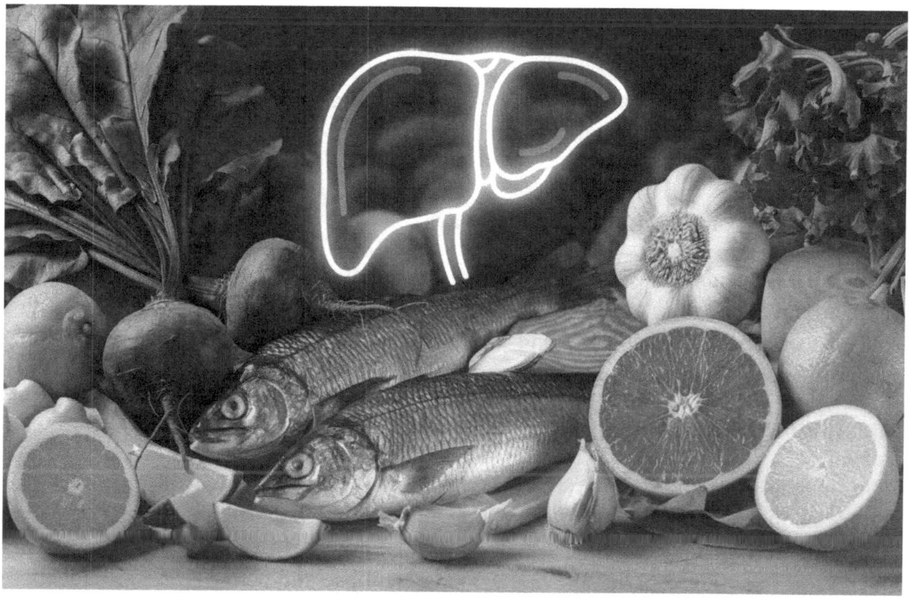

Liver regeneration is a remarkable process, but it does not happen in isolation. The liver needs a constant supply of specific nutrients to repair damaged tissue, reduce inflammation, and maintain healthy metabolic function.

1. Essential Nutrients for Liver Repair and Regeneration

A nutrient-rich fatty liver diet plan does more than support detoxification. It also creates the building blocks the liver uses to rebuild itself.

When these nutrients are consistently provided, the liver can reverse fatty liver changes more effectively and protect itself from future damage.

Protein for Tissue Repair

Adequate protein is vital for regenerating liver tissue. Amino acids are required for the production of enzymes, structural proteins, and antioxidants like glutathione. Without enough protein, healing slows and detoxification pathways can become less efficient. High-quality sources include fish, poultry, legumes, eggs, and, for those who tolerate dairy, yogurt or kefir with live cultures.

Healthy Fats for Anti-Inflammatory Support

Not all fats are harmful. Healthy fats from sources such as extra virgin olive oil, avocados, walnuts, chia seeds, flaxseeds, and fatty fish reduce liver inflammation and improve cell membrane integrity. These fats are essential for absorbing fat-soluble vitamins like A, D, E, and K, which are needed for optimal liver function.

Antioxidants for Cellular Protection

Oxidative stress is a major driver of liver cell damage. Antioxidants neutralize free radicals before they can harm tissue. Vitamin C from citrus fruits, strawberries, and bell peppers supports collagen formation and immune function. Vitamin E from almonds, sunflower seeds, and spinach helps protect fatty structures in cells. Selenium, found in Brazil nuts and seafood, supports the production of glutathione, the liver's master antioxidant.

B Vitamins for Energy and Detox Pathways

B vitamins, especially B2, B3, B6, B9, and B12, play a direct role in liver metabolism and detoxification. They are involved in converting food into energy, processing amino acids, and supporting phase one and phase two detox pathways. Leafy greens, whole grains, eggs, and lean meats are rich sources.

Minerals for Enzyme Function

Zinc, magnesium, and copper are essential for the enzymes involved in liver repair and metabolism. Zinc aids in tissue healing and immune balance, magnesium supports hundreds of enzymatic processes including those for energy production, and copper plays a role in antioxidant defense. Nuts, seeds, shellfish, and whole grains provide these minerals in bioavailable forms.

Phytonutrients for Anti-Inflammatory Action

Plant compounds such as polyphenols and flavonoids help reduce liver inflammation and improve blood vessel health. They are found in berries, green tea, dark leafy greens, and herbs like rosemary and oregano. Incorporating these regularly helps maintain a steady anti-inflammatory environment for liver healing.

Integrating Nutrients into a Fatty Liver Diet Plan

A single meal cannot provide all the nutrients needed for liver regeneration, but a well-planned week of eating can. For example:

- Breakfast might include oatmeal topped with blueberries, chia seeds, and walnuts.
- Lunch could be a quinoa salad with leafy greens, chickpeas, olive oil, and lemon.
- Dinner might be grilled salmon with steamed broccoli and roasted sweet potatoes.

This balance of proteins, healthy fats, complex carbohydrates, and colorful vegetables ensures the liver receives what it needs to heal.

2. The Role of Intermittent Fasting in Liver Recovery

Intermittent fasting is not about extreme deprivation but about creating periods when the body is not processing food. These fasting windows allow the liver to shift focus from digesting and storing nutrients to repairing tissue, processing stored fat, and improving metabolic flexibility.

The most common approaches are the 16:8 method, where eating is restricted to an eight-hour window each day, and the 5:2 method, where calorie intake is reduced on two days per week while eating normally on the others.

Benefits for Fatty Liver and Inflammation

Research shows intermittent fasting can help reduce liver fat, improve insulin sensitivity, and lower markers of inflammation. By giving the liver extended breaks from processing constant glucose and fat intake, fasting helps it mobilize stored fat for energy. This process is particularly beneficial in reversing fatty liver and reducing liver inflammation.

Improved Insulin Sensitivity

Insulin resistance is a key factor in the development of non-alcoholic fatty liver disease. Intermittent fasting lowers fasting insulin levels, which helps cells respond more effectively to insulin's signals. Improved insulin sensitivity means less glucose is stored as fat in the liver.

Supporting Detox Pathways During Fasting

During fasting periods, the liver continues its detox work, breaking down and removing stored toxins. To support this process, hydration is essential. Herbal teas, plain water, and mineral-rich broths can help maintain electrolyte balance and keep bile flow healthy.

Unlike restrictive cleanses, intermittent fasting does not deprive the liver of essential nutrients because meals during eating windows can be nutrient-dense and supportive.

Cautions and Considerations

Intermittent fasting is not suitable for everyone. People with certain medical conditions, those who are pregnant or breastfeeding, and individuals on specific medications should consult a healthcare provider before starting. It is also important not to use fasting as an excuse to eat nutrient-poor, processed foods during eating periods, as this will undermine liver recovery.

Combining Fasting with an Anti-Inflammatory Diet

The real benefits of intermittent fasting for liver regeneration come when it is paired with a nutrient-rich, anti-inflammatory diet. Meals should emphasize vegetables, lean protein, healthy fats, and low-glycemic carbohydrates. This combination helps reduce liver inflammation, stabilize blood sugar, and provide the building blocks for repair.

An Example of a Supportive Intermittent Fasting Day

- Morning: Herbal tea or water with lemon during fasting window
- Midday (first meal): Grilled chicken salad with leafy greens, avocado, olive oil, and pumpkin seeds
- Late afternoon snack: Greek yogurt with berries and flaxseed

- Evening (final meal): Baked cod with quinoa, steamed asparagus, and a side of roasted carrots

This schedule gives the liver a solid fasting period overnight and into the morning while delivering a nutrient-dense intake during eating hours.

3. Building a Fatty Liver Diet Plan for Life

Short-term diets may help reduce liver fat temporarily, but fatty liver disease can return if old eating habits resume. A sustainable fatty liver diet plan should be built around realistic, enjoyable foods that can be maintained for years. This is not just about reducing fat in the liver but also supporting overall health, improving digestion, reducing inflammation, and ensuring nutrient sufficiency for liver regeneration.

Balancing Macronutrients for Liver Health

A successful long-term plan provides balanced amounts of protein, carbohydrates, and healthy fats. Protein supports tissue repair and detox enzymes. Complex carbohydrates from whole grains, legumes, and vegetables provide slow-releasing energy without causing sharp blood sugar spikes. Healthy fats, especially those rich in omega-3s, help reduce liver inflammation and improve fat metabolism.

Instead of aiming for strict macronutrient percentages, focus on including all three in every meal. This stabilizes blood sugar, keeps energy steady, and prevents overloading the liver with one type of nutrient.

Making Vegetables the Foundation

Vegetables should form the largest portion of most meals. They supply antioxidants, vitamins, minerals, and fiber that support both liver and digestive health. Leafy greens, cruciferous vegetables, brightly colored peppers, and root vegetables all contribute to reducing oxidative stress and improving detoxification.

To make this habit sustainable, rotate vegetables weekly to avoid taste fatigue and ensure a broad spectrum of nutrients.

Protein Choices for Fatty Liver Recovery

High-quality protein helps maintain muscle mass, which is important for metabolic health. It also supports the production of liver enzymes and antioxidants. Fish, skinless poultry, eggs, beans, lentils, and low-fat dairy can all be part of the plan. For variety, include plant-based proteins like quinoa or tempeh.

Managing Carbohydrates the Right Way

Carbohydrates are not the enemy, but refined versions can quickly lead to fat storage in the liver. Choosing whole grains, legumes, and starchy vegetables ensures fiber intake stays high, slowing the release of glucose into the blood. This helps reverse insulin resistance, a key factor in fatty liver disease.

Healthy Fats for Anti-Inflammatory Support

Avocados, olive oil, walnuts, chia seeds, and flaxseeds provide fats that protect cell membranes and help regulate inflammation. Limit processed oils and deep-fried foods, which can increase oxidative stress and hinder liver regeneration.

Portion Control Without Restriction

A fatty liver diet plan for life should not feel overly restrictive. Rather than cutting out entire food groups, the focus should be on portion awareness. Eating until satisfied instead of overly full reduces the digestive load and helps the liver process nutrients more efficiently.

Adapting the Plan for Different Life Stages

The core principles of a liver-friendly eating pattern remain the same, but calorie needs and nutrient priorities may shift with age, activity level, and health status. Regular check-ins with a healthcare professional can help tailor the plan as needed.

4. Energy-Boosting Foods that Improve Digestion Naturally

When digestion is sluggish, energy levels drop. The body spends more time and resources breaking down food, leaving less energy available for daily activities. Poor digestion can also mean fewer nutrients reach the bloodstream, which limits what the liver and other organs can use for repair and regeneration. By choosing foods that improve digestion naturally, you also enhance your ability to maintain steady energy throughout the day.

Whole Foods That Support Digestive Efficiency

Some foods work double duty by promoting healthy digestion while also providing an energy boost.

- **Oats** deliver soluble fiber that feeds beneficial gut bacteria and helps maintain stable blood sugar.
- **Leafy greens** like spinach and kale supply magnesium, which supports muscle relaxation in the digestive tract.
- **Bananas** provide easily digestible carbohydrates and potassium, which helps regulate fluid balance and nerve function.
- **Berries** are rich in antioxidants and fiber without being heavy on the digestive system.
- **Fermented foods** like yogurt, kefir, sauerkraut, and kimchi replenish probiotics, aiding gut-liver balance.

Energizing Proteins That Are Easy to Digest

Eggs, fish, and skinless poultry are lighter proteins that supply amino acids without overburdening the digestive system. For plant-based eaters, lentils and tempeh are good choices, though they should be introduced gradually if digestion is sensitive.

Healthy Fats That Keep Energy Steady

Medium-chain triglycerides (MCTs) from coconut oil are quickly absorbed and used as a direct energy source. Nuts and seeds provide lasting fuel while also delivering minerals and anti-inflammatory fats. Including small amounts of healthy fat with each meal helps maintain satiety and energy balance.

Hydration as an Energy Factor

Even mild dehydration can cause fatigue and sluggish digestion. Water helps move food through the digestive tract and aids in nutrient absorption. Herbal teas such as peppermint or ginger can soothe the stomach and stimulate digestion, contributing to both comfort and energy.

Spices and Herbs for Digestive and Energy Support

Certain spices not only enhance flavor but also aid digestion and circulation. Ginger can improve gastric emptying and reduce nausea. Turmeric offers anti-inflammatory benefits that support the liver. Cinnamon helps regulate blood sugar, reducing energy crashes after meals.

Meal Timing and Energy Rhythm

Energy dips often follow large, heavy meals that take a long time to digest. Eating smaller, balanced meals at regular intervals can prevent these crashes. Including a mix of protein, healthy fats, and complex carbohydrates at each meal keeps digestion steady and energy levels stable.

Listening to the Body's Responses

Foods that energize one person may make another feel sluggish, depending on digestion and metabolism. Tracking meals and energy levels can help identify patterns. Adjusting the diet based on these observations ensures it remains both supportive of digestion and sustainable for liver health.

5. Hydration and Liver Health — The Right Way to Drink Water

Water is the foundation of every detox process in the body, and the liver depends on it for nearly all of its functions. It is the medium in which nutrients travel, toxins are diluted, and waste products are carried to the kidneys and intestines for elimination. Without adequate hydration, the liver must work harder to process and remove compounds from the blood, which can slow recovery in conditions like fatty liver disease.

Good hydration also supports bile production, which is essential for breaking down fats and carrying fat-soluble toxins out of the body. A fatty liver diet plan that neglects hydration will struggle to deliver the full benefits of its nutrient-dense foods.

How Dehydration Affects the Liver

When the body lacks water, blood becomes more concentrated, which makes it harder for the liver to filter waste efficiently. This can increase oxidative stress, a known contributor to liver inflammation. Dehydration also thickens bile, making it less effective in fat digestion and potentially leading to sluggish digestion and nutrient malabsorption.

The Right Way to Hydrate for Liver Health

Hydration doesn't just consider the total amount of water consumed, but also how and when it is consumed. Large amounts of water all at once may pass quickly through the system without effectively rehydrating tissues. Smaller, consistent sips throughout the day keep hydration steady and support constant liver function.

Factors That Influence Hydration Needs

Everyone's optimal intake varies depending on body size, activity level, climate, and dietary composition. High-protein and high-fiber diets can require more water to process nutrients efficiently. Those living in hot or dry climates or engaging in regular exercise need to be especially mindful of replacing fluids.

Beverages That Support Liver Regeneration

Plain water is best, but herbal teas like dandelion, ginger, or green tea can offer additional antioxidant and digestive benefits. Infusing water with lemon, cucumber, or fresh herbs can make it more appealing and provide small amounts of vitamins and phytonutrients. Coconut water, in moderation, can help restore electrolytes without excess sugar.

Beverages to Limit or Avoid

Sugary drinks, sodas, and excessive fruit juice can raise blood sugar and triglyceride levels, contributing to fat accumulation in the liver. Energy drinks and excessive caffeine can also stress the liver, especially when hydration is already poor. Alcohol, even in small amounts, places an immediate detox burden on the liver and should be avoided entirely for those aiming to reverse fatty liver.

Hydration Tips for Better Digestion and Energy

Drinking a glass of water shortly after waking helps replenish fluids lost overnight and stimulates gentle bile flow. Having small amounts of water 20 to 30 minutes before meals can aid digestion, while excessive water during meals may dilute digestive enzymes. Hydrating between meals rather than during them often improves digestion for those with bloating or sluggish stomach emptying.

6. Planning Meals for Maximum Nutrient Absorption

A nutrient-rich fatty liver diet plan is only effective if the body can absorb and utilize those nutrients. Poor absorption can occur when digestion is compromised, bile flow is inadequate, or certain foods are combined in ways that block nutrient uptake.

Optimizing meals for absorption ensures that every bite delivers maximum benefit for liver regeneration and overall health.

The Role of Healthy Fats in Nutrient Uptake

Many vitamins and phytonutrients are fat-soluble, meaning they require dietary fat to be absorbed. Vitamins A, D, E, and K, as well as carotenoids from colorful vegetables, need healthy fats like olive oil, avocado, nuts, or seeds in the same meal for proper absorption. A salad with olive oil dressing, for example, will provide more usable nutrients than one eaten dry.

Pairing Foods for Better Absorption

Certain nutrients are absorbed more effectively when paired with complementary foods.

- Vitamin C from citrus or bell peppers enhances the absorption of iron from plant sources such as lentils or spinach.
- Zinc absorption from legumes improves when they are soaked before cooking to reduce phytate content.
- Calcium from leafy greens is better absorbed when the oxalate content is lowered by lightly steaming the vegetables.

Meal Timing and Digestive Energy

Spacing meals evenly throughout the day helps maintain stable blood sugar and energy while giving the digestive system time to process each intake fully. Eating too frequently can overload digestion, while skipping meals can lead to overeating later, which strains the liver.

Reducing Inhibitors of Nutrient Absorption

Some compounds in food can interfere with nutrient uptake if consumed in excess. Phytates in raw grains and legumes, oxalates in spinach and beet greens, and tannins in tea and coffee can all reduce mineral absorption. These effects can be minimized through soaking, sprouting, fermenting, and cooking foods appropriately.

Including Fermented Foods for Digestive Support

Fermented foods like sauerkraut, kimchi, kefir, and miso can introduce beneficial bacteria into the gut, improving digestion and enhancing nutrient absorption. A healthier gut microbiome also reduces the inflammatory load on the liver.

Portion Balance and Digestive Comfort

Meals that are too large can slow stomach emptying and reduce nutrient uptake efficiency. Smaller, balanced meals allow for better breakdown of food and steadier delivery of nutrients into the bloodstream. For those aiming to improve digestion naturally and reduce liver inflammation, portion control is as important as food quality.

Practical Meal Planning for Liver Healing

For breakfast, a vegetable omelet with avocado and a side of berries provides protein, healthy fats, and antioxidants. Lunch could be quinoa with grilled salmon, steamed broccoli, and olive oil. Dinner might include lentil soup with a mixed green salad topped with pumpkin seeds and lemon-tahini dressing. Snacks can be Greek yogurt with flaxseed or a handful of walnuts with sliced apple. Each of these examples combines nutrient-dense foods in ways that maximize absorption and support both digestion and liver health.

Chapter 10: The Most Effective Supplements for Liver Support

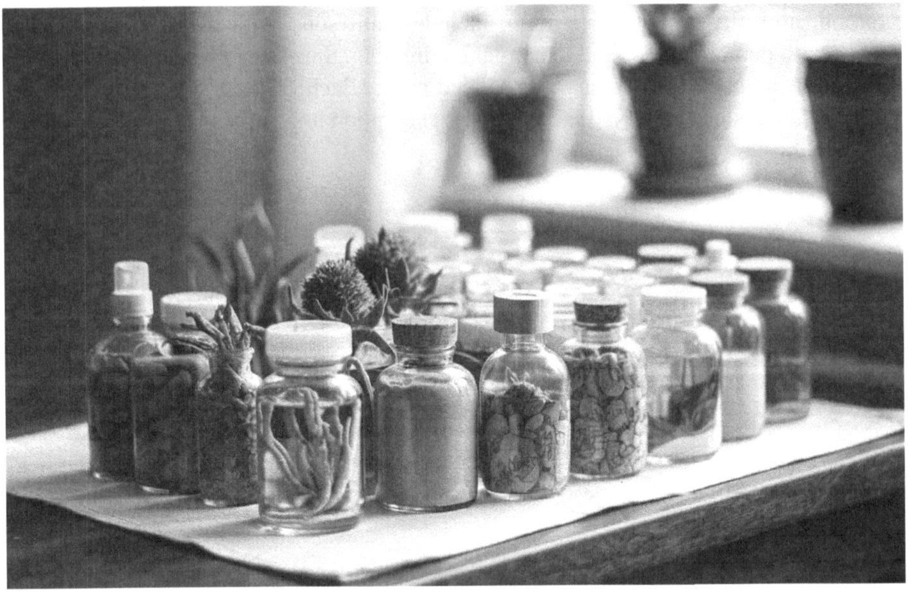

A healthy liver is central to energy production, digestion, detoxification, and overall metabolic balance. For those aiming to reverse fatty liver, reduce liver inflammation, and protect against future damage, nutrition and lifestyle form the foundation. However, targeted supplementation and herbal support can provide an extra layer of protection and accelerate regeneration.

1. Powerful Supplements and Herbs for Liver Regeneration

Milk Thistle for Liver Cell Protection and Regeneration

Milk thistle (***Silybum marianum***) is one of the most widely researched herbal supplements for liver health. Its active compound, silymarin, has antioxidant, anti-inflammatory, and membrane-stabilizing properties. Silymarin works by neutralizing free radicals that contribute to liver cell damage and by promoting protein synthesis, which aids in the regeneration of liver tissue.

Several clinical studies suggest milk thistle can help improve liver enzyme levels in people with fatty liver disease and other chronic liver conditions. While it is not a replacement for a fatty liver diet plan or lifestyle changes, it can serve as an additional protective measure.

N-Acetyl Cysteine (NAC) for Glutathione Support

NAC is a form of the amino acid cysteine and is best known for boosting the body's production of glutathione, the liver's most important antioxidant. Glutathione plays a key role in phase two detoxification, where toxins are neutralized and prepared for elimination. Without sufficient glutathione, toxins can accumulate, leading to oxidative stress and inflammation in the liver.

NAC supplementation has been studied for its ability to reduce liver inflammation, improve enzyme levels, and protect against damage from environmental toxins, alcohol, and certain medications. It is often used in clinical settings for acute liver toxicity, which speaks to its potency.

Curcumin for Reducing Inflammation and Supporting Bile Flow

Curcumin, the primary active compound in turmeric, has strong anti-inflammatory and antioxidant effects. It helps regulate inflammatory pathways, reduces oxidative stress, and promotes healthy bile flow, which supports fat digestion and the removal of fat-soluble toxins.

Research on curcumin and fatty liver disease shows that it can help reduce liver fat content, improve liver enzyme profiles, and support metabolic health. Its absorption is enhanced when taken with black pepper extract (piperine) or consumed with a source of healthy fat such as olive oil or avocado.

When to Consider These Supplements

These three supplements can be particularly helpful for people looking to reverse fatty liver, reduce liver inflammation, and protect against further damage. They work best when used alongside an anti-inflammatory diet, regular physical activity, and other natural remedies for liver health.

It is important to choose high-quality products from reputable companies, as supplements are not regulated as strictly as medications. Third-party testing for purity and potency is recommended.

Cautions and Interactions

While generally safe, each of these supplements may interact with certain medications. Milk thistle can affect drug metabolism in the liver. NAC may interact with nitroglycerin, and curcumin can thin the blood, which is relevant for people taking anticoagulants. Consultation with a healthcare provider before starting any supplement regimen is essential.

Dandelion Root for Gentle Liver Support

Dandelion root has a long history in traditional medicine as a liver tonic. It is believed to stimulate bile production, which aids in fat digestion and helps move toxins out of the liver and digestive tract. Dandelion root also contains antioxidants that may help protect liver cells from oxidative damage.

It can be consumed as a tea, tincture, or capsule. For those aiming to improve digestion naturally while supporting liver health, dandelion tea before meals can be a gentle addition.

Artichoke Leaf for Detox and Cholesterol Balance

Artichoke leaf extract supports liver function by increasing bile production and improving cholesterol metabolism. It contains compounds such as cynarin, which have been studied for their potential to lower LDL cholesterol and improve fat digestion. This is particularly relevant for people with fatty liver disease, where cholesterol balance and bile flow are often compromised.

Artichoke leaf is available as a supplement or in dried form for tea. It pairs well with a fatty liver diet plan that emphasizes whole foods and anti-inflammatory ingredients.

Other Beneficial Herbs for Liver Regeneration

Several other herbs can be included in a comprehensive liver health guide:

- **Schisandra berry** is an adaptogen used in traditional Chinese medicine to protect liver cells and enhance detoxification enzymes.
- **Ginger root** improves digestion and circulation, indirectly benefiting liver function.
- **Peppermint leaf** can relax the digestive tract, easing bile flow and reducing discomfort from poor fat digestion.
- **Burdock root** supports detox through both the liver and the skin, helping remove waste products.

These herbs can be rotated or blended into herbal teas, offering a natural remedy approach that is gentle enough for long-term use.

How to Incorporate These Herbs into Daily Life

Herbal teas are one of the easiest ways to introduce liver-supportive plants into a daily routine. A morning cup of dandelion and ginger tea or an evening blend of peppermint and schisandra can provide ongoing benefits without overwhelming the liver. For those who prefer supplements, standardized extracts can deliver more concentrated doses.

When adding herbs, it is important to start with small amounts to observe tolerance, especially for those with sensitive digestion.

Combining Supplements and Herbs for Synergy

Using milk thistle, NAC, curcumin, and supportive herbs together can create a comprehensive plan for liver regeneration. Each works on different aspects of liver health, from reducing inflammation and oxidative stress to improving bile flow and nutrient absorption. This synergistic approach can make a significant difference for those working to reverse fatty liver and reduce liver inflammation.

2. Choosing High-Quality Supplements Safely

The supplement industry is not regulated in the same way as prescription medications, which means the quality, purity, and potency of products can vary widely. For someone aiming to reverse fatty liver, reduce liver inflammation, or support liver regeneration, using poor-quality supplements can be ineffective at best and harmful at worst. Contaminants, fillers, and inaccurate labeling are not uncommon in low-quality products, making careful selection essential.

Looking for Third-Party Testing

Reputable supplement brands often submit their products to independent labs for third-party testing. This process verifies that the product contains what is stated on the label and is free from harmful contaminants such as heavy metals, pesticides, or harmful microbes. Seals from organizations like USP (United States Pharmacopeia), NSF International, or ConsumerLab can indicate higher quality standards.

Checking for Standardized Extracts

When using herbal supplements as natural remedies for liver health, it is important to choose products with standardized extracts. This ensures a consistent level of active compounds, such as silymarin in milk thistle or curcumin in turmeric. Without standardization, the potency can vary from batch to batch, making it difficult to achieve consistent benefits.

Avoiding Unnecessary Additives

Many low-cost supplements contain artificial colors, flavors, or fillers that do not contribute to liver healing and may even burden detox pathways. While small amounts may not cause harm, they are not necessary for an effective liver health guide. Choosing supplements with minimal, clean ingredient lists helps avoid these unnecessary extras.

Verifying the Source of Ingredients

Supplements derived from high-quality raw materials tend to be more effective and safer. For example, fish oil supplements should come from sustainably sourced fish and be purified to remove mercury and other toxins. Plant-based supplements should be free from pesticide residues and ideally sourced from organically grown plants.

Reputation and Transparency of the Brand

A brand's track record says a lot about its reliability. Established companies that invest in research, publish testing results, and provide detailed product information are generally safer choices. Transparent labeling and responsive customer service are indicators that a company values consumer trust.

When to Seek Professional Guidance

Even high-quality supplements can cause interactions with medications or medical conditions. Consulting with a healthcare provider familiar with both conventional medicine and natural remedies for liver health can prevent unwanted effects. This is especially important for people with chronic conditions, those taking multiple medications, or anyone using higher-potency supplements for targeted results.

3. Timing and Dosages for Maximum Benefit

Why Timing Matters in Supplement Use

Supplements for liver regeneration and fatty liver reversal can be more effective when taken at specific times of day or with certain foods. The timing can influence absorption, interaction with other nutrients, and the way the body processes active compounds. Poor timing may lead to reduced benefits or mild digestive discomfort, which can discourage consistent use.

Fat-Soluble vs. Water-Soluble Compounds

Some supplements are better absorbed with meals containing healthy fats, while others work best on an empty stomach.

- Fat-soluble nutrients, such as vitamin E or curcumin, should be taken with a meal that contains olive oil, avocado, or nuts to improve absorption.
- Water-soluble compounds, like vitamin C or NAC, can be taken with or without food, but timing them between meals may reduce competition with other nutrients for absorption.

Splitting Doses for Steady Support

For certain nutrients, splitting the daily dosage into two or three smaller amounts can provide more consistent blood levels throughout the day. This approach may be beneficial for liver-supportive antioxidants and some herbal remedies, allowing for ongoing delivery of protective compounds.

Coordinating with Meals for Better Tolerance

Some people experience mild stomach upset when taking supplements on an empty stomach, particularly with herbs like milk thistle or artichoke leaf. Taking these with meals can improve tolerance and still provide effective absorption. For example, incorporating them into a midday or evening meal as part of a fatty liver diet plan ensures the body is nourished while supplements do their work.

Avoiding Interference Between Supplements

Certain supplements can compete for absorption or alter the effectiveness of others if taken together. For example, high doses of calcium can interfere with zinc and magnesium uptake. Separating these by a few hours ensures better utilization of each nutrient. Similarly, some herbal extracts with strong antioxidant effects may reduce the potency of certain medications, making it important to plan timing carefully.

Considering the Body's Natural Rhythms

The liver follows a circadian rhythm, performing specific functions more actively at certain times of day. Detoxification and repair processes are often most active during the evening and overnight. Taking liver-supportive supplements in the afternoon or early evening may align with these natural cycles, although this can vary based on individual needs and the type of supplement.

Adjusting Dosages Based on Goals and Response

Dosage recommendations on supplement labels are general guidelines and may not be ideal for every person. Factors such as body weight, metabolism, diet quality, and the severity of liver issues can influence how much is needed. Starting with the lowest effective dose and gradually increasing under professional supervision allows for personalized fine-tuning.

Consistency for Lasting Results

No supplement can reverse fatty liver or reduce liver inflammation overnight. Benefits build over time with regular use, particularly when paired with an anti-inflammatory diet and healthy lifestyle habits. Skipping doses occasionally will not undo progress, but consistent intake provides the steady support the liver needs for regeneration.

4. Supplements for Reducing Liver Fat and Inflammation

While diet and lifestyle changes are the foundation of a successful fatty liver reversal strategy, certain supplements can accelerate progress by addressing specific imbalances in fat metabolism and inflammation. Supplements for this purpose often work by improving insulin sensitivity, enhancing fat breakdown, and providing antioxidant support to protect liver cells from further damage. When used wisely, they can complement the fatty liver diet plan and help the body reach a healthier balance faster.

Omega-3 Fatty Acids for Fat Reduction

Omega-3 fatty acids from fish oil, algal oil, or krill oil are among the most researched nutrients for reducing liver fat. They help regulate triglyceride levels, improve insulin sensitivity, and reduce inflammatory markers in people with fatty liver disease. These fats are incorporated into cell membranes, making them more flexible and less prone to oxidative damage. Regular supplementation can also help balance the ratio of omega-3 to omega-6 fats, which is crucial for reducing inflammation.

Vitamin E for Antioxidant Protection

Vitamin E is a fat-soluble antioxidant that protects liver cells from oxidative stress. In certain studies, it has been shown to improve liver enzyme levels and reduce signs of inflammation in people with non-alcoholic steatohepatitis. However, dosage and duration should be monitored closely, as excessive intake can have risks. A healthcare professional should guide supplementation to ensure safety.

N-Acetyl Cysteine (NAC) for Glutathione Support

NAC boosts the body's production of glutathione, the primary antioxidant responsible for neutralizing harmful compounds in the liver. This helps reduce oxidative stress, which is a key driver of inflammation in fatty liver disease. NAC supplementation can also improve detoxification pathways, allowing the liver to focus more on regeneration.

Berberine for Metabolic Health

Berberine is a plant-derived compound that has been shown to improve insulin sensitivity, lower blood sugar, and reduce liver fat accumulation. Its effects on metabolism make it particularly valuable for people with fatty liver linked to insulin resistance or metabolic syndrome.

Curcumin for Inflammation Control

Curcumin, the active component in turmeric, has strong anti-inflammatory and antioxidant properties. It can help reduce inflammatory pathways and improve bile flow, which supports the removal of fat-soluble toxins. Combining curcumin with black pepper extract can improve its absorption and enhance its effects.

Practical Use in a Liver Health Guide

These supplements work best when introduced gradually and in combination with an anti-inflammatory diet rich in vegetables, lean proteins, and healthy fats. They should be chosen based on individual needs and used under the guidance of a healthcare professional to avoid interactions with medications or excessive nutrient intake.

5. Synergy Between Food and Supplements

Supplements are not meant to replace food but to work alongside it. Whole foods supply a broad range of nutrients, fiber, and phytonutrients that cannot be fully replicated in capsule form. Supplements, on the other hand, can provide concentrated doses of specific compounds that might be difficult to get in adequate amounts through diet alone. When both are aligned, they can create a more powerful and sustainable approach to reverse fatty liver and reduce liver inflammation.

Food as the Foundation

A nutrient-rich diet provides the baseline for liver regeneration. Foods such as leafy greens, cruciferous vegetables, berries, citrus fruits, legumes, and fatty fish deliver a mix of antioxidants, vitamins, and minerals. These help maintain healthy liver function, balance blood sugar, and improve digestion naturally. Without this base, supplements have less impact because the body is still lacking the broad spectrum of nutrients it needs for repair.

Enhancing Food Benefits with Supplements

Some supplements can boost the effects of nutrient-rich foods by improving absorption or delivering higher concentrations of active compounds. For example:

- Taking curcumin with a meal that includes healthy fats can improve its bioavailability.

- Pairing vitamin C-rich foods like bell peppers with iron-rich plant foods like lentils improves iron absorption, which supports oxygen delivery to tissues.
- Combining probiotics with prebiotic-rich foods like garlic and onions enhances gut microbiome diversity, which reduces inflammatory stress on the liver.

Meal Timing and Supplement Use

Certain supplements are best taken with food to improve absorption, while others may work better on an empty stomach. Fat-soluble vitamins such as vitamin E and omega-3 fatty acids should be consumed alongside a meal containing healthy fats. NAC, on the other hand, can be taken between meals for optimal uptake. Understanding these timing considerations ensures the nutrients from both food and supplements are fully utilized.

Reducing Overlap and Avoiding Excess

Some people make the mistake of doubling up on nutrients by taking multiple supplements that contain the same ingredient. For example, fish oil capsules combined with a high daily intake of oily fish can push omega-3 intake beyond recommended levels. The same can happen with antioxidants like vitamin E or herbal extracts. Careful planning prevents unnecessary excess and reduces the risk of nutrient imbalances.

Examples of Synergy in Practice

- A lunch of grilled salmon, steamed broccoli, and quinoa, combined with a fish oil supplement, maximizes omega-3 intake for reducing liver inflammation.
- A smoothie with spinach, berries, chia seeds, and almond butter provides antioxidants and fiber, while an added curcumin capsule enhances anti-inflammatory benefits.
- A dinner of lentil stew and mixed greens, followed by a probiotic supplement, strengthens gut health and supports the gut–liver connection.

Maintaining Consistency for Long-Term Results

The synergy between food and supplements works best when maintained over the long term. Short bursts of supplementation without dietary support rarely lead to lasting changes in liver health. A well-balanced fatty liver diet plan, supported by carefully chosen supplements, creates an environment where the liver can regenerate, reduce inflammation, and improve metabolic function consistently.

Chapter 11: The Lifestyle Blueprint for a Healthy Liver

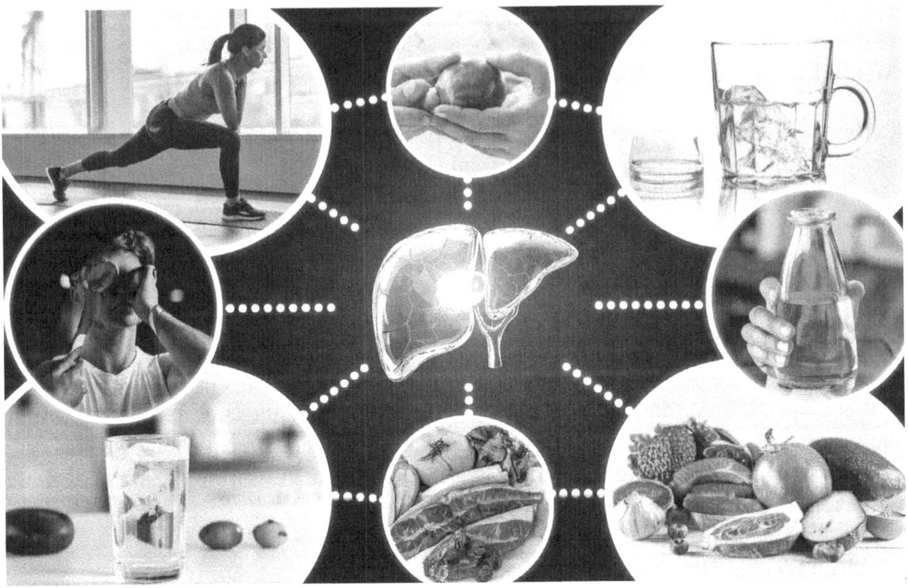

1. Sleep and Circadian Rhythms and Their Importance for Liver Health

Sleep is not just rest for the mind; it is one of the most active times for the liver. During the night, the liver carries out vital processes such as detoxification, nutrient metabolism, and tissue repair. The body's circadian rhythm, which governs the natural 24-hour cycle of physiological processes, has a profound influence on how effectively the liver performs these tasks. When sleep schedules are irregular, or when rest is insufficient, the rhythm can be disrupted, reducing the efficiency of liver regeneration.

Aiming for seven to nine hours of quality sleep each night allows the liver to complete its overnight repair cycle. Consistency is key. Going to bed and waking up at the same time daily helps reinforce the body's internal clock, which in turn helps regulate hormone release, metabolism, and detoxification processes. This stability supports long-term goals such as reversing fatty liver and reducing liver inflammation.

Practical steps to improve sleep quality include creating a dark, cool sleeping environment, limiting screen exposure in the hour before bed, and avoiding heavy meals close to bedtime. Evening routines such as herbal teas, light stretching, or calming breathing exercises can also help signal to the body that it is time to rest.

2. The Impact of Stress on Liver Function and Stress Management Techniques

Stress can affect the liver in ways that are both direct and indirect. Elevated stress hormones such as cortisol can increase blood sugar levels, which over time contributes to fat storage in the liver. Chronic stress also promotes systemic inflammation, which can slow liver regeneration and make it harder to reverse fatty liver.

When stress is prolonged, the immune system can become imbalanced, increasing the risk of inflammation-related damage to liver cells. Stress also influences lifestyle habits. People under strain may gravitate toward processed foods, skip exercise, or rely on alcohol, all of which put additional pressure on the liver.

To protect liver health, stress management needs to be an ongoing part of a fatty liver diet plan. This does not necessarily require long meditation sessions or complex programs. Simple, consistent practices are often the most effective. Walking outdoors, spending time in nature, or engaging in a creative hobby can help lower stress levels.

Breathing techniques can also be powerful tools. For example, slow, deep breathing for five minutes can reduce cortisol levels and improve circulation. Gentle yoga or tai chi combines movement with mindfulness, supporting both mental balance and physical circulation, which benefits the liver. Social connections matter as well; speaking with friends, family, or a supportive group can reduce the mental burden of stress.

3. The Best and Worst Types of Exercise for Liver Health

Movement is one of the most reliable ways to improve liver function and speed the reversal of fatty liver. Exercise improves insulin sensitivity, reduces fat storage in the liver, and helps control body weight. The best approach combines both aerobic and resistance training to maximize benefits for metabolic health and liver regeneration.

Aerobic exercises such as brisk walking, cycling, swimming, or light jogging can help reduce liver fat and improve circulation. Aiming for at least 150 minutes per week of moderate-intensity aerobic activity is a good target for most adults. Resistance training, which can be done with weights, resistance bands, or bodyweight exercises, builds muscle mass. This is important because muscle tissue increases resting metabolism, helping the body burn more calories even at rest.

High-intensity interval training (HIIT) can also be beneficial in small doses, as it improves cardiovascular health and insulin sensitivity in a short period of time. However, it is important to progress gradually to avoid fatigue or injury, especially for those just beginning an exercise routine after a period of inactivity.

Some forms of exercise can hinder liver healing if overdone. Excessive endurance training without adequate recovery may increase oxidative stress and inflammation, placing an additional burden on the liver. Exercise routines that lead to frequent dehydration or nutrient depletion, such as extreme heat-based workouts without proper hydration, should be approached with caution.

The key is finding a balance that supports the liver without overstressing it. Pairing regular exercise with an anti-inflammatory diet, proper hydration, and adequate sleep creates a strong foundation for long-term liver health.

4. Creating a Metabolic Reset Program for Long-Term Results

A metabolic reset program is not a quick fix. It is a structured approach that helps the body switch from storing excess calories as fat to using them efficiently for energy. For those aiming to reverse fatty liver, this shift is essential. The program should integrate nutrition, movement, and recovery into a balanced rhythm that the body can maintain long-term.

Nutritionally, the focus remains on an anti-inflammatory diet that is rich in vegetables, lean proteins, healthy fats, and low-glycemic carbohydrates. Meal timing plays a role as well. Avoiding constant snacking allows insulin levels to stabilize, which helps reduce fat storage in the liver. Some people benefit from a gentle form of intermittent fasting, such as a 12-hour overnight fast, to encourage fat metabolism without causing energy crashes.

Physical activity is a core part of the reset. Combining resistance training with moderate aerobic exercise improves muscle-to-fat ratio and keeps metabolism active. Recovery days are equally important, allowing the liver to focus on regeneration rather than processing the byproducts of intense exercise.

Tracking progress is part of the program. This can be as simple as noting energy levels, sleep quality, digestion, and mood alongside body measurements or periodic blood work. Over time, these markers reveal whether the plan is moving you toward improved metabolic balance and better liver health.

5. Building Sustainable Habits for Liver Wellness

Lasting liver regeneration comes from consistency, not perfection. Sustainable habits are those that fit into daily life without feeling like a burden. The goal is to make liver-friendly choices so routine that they require little thought.

One effective method is habit stacking, which is pairing a new behavior with an existing one. For example, if you already drink a glass of water in the morning, you might add a handful of leafy greens to your breakfast or take a short walk afterward. Small, repeated actions are more likely to stick than large, sudden changes.

Preparation is another pillar of sustainability. Keeping the kitchen stocked with ingredients for quick, liver-friendly meals prevents reliance on processed or fast foods. Cooking in batches, prepping vegetables ahead of time, and having healthy snacks ready can help maintain momentum.

Mindful eating is a habit that supports both digestion and liver function. Taking time to chew food thoroughly, avoiding distractions during meals, and stopping when comfortably satisfied reduces strain on the digestive system and allows the liver to process nutrients more effectively.

6. Motivation and Mindset for Healing

Mindset often determines whether lifestyle changes last. Many people begin a fatty liver diet plan with enthusiasm but lose focus when results slow or life becomes busy. Understanding that liver healing is a gradual process can prevent frustration and help maintain motivation.

One useful approach is to set process-based goals rather than outcome-only goals. Instead of focusing solely on reducing liver fat by a certain percentage, commit to walking five days a week, cooking most meals at home, or incorporating leafy greens into two meals a day. These actions are within your control and will naturally lead to measurable improvements over time.

Celebrating progress, even small changes like improved digestion, steadier energy, or better sleep, reinforces positive behavior. Keeping a journal of these wins can be a reminder of how far you have come, especially on days when motivation dips.

Support from friends, family, or a health coach can also help maintain commitment. Having someone to share progress with or to hold you accountable makes it easier to keep going, even during challenging periods. Over time, these lifestyle changes become ingrained, and maintaining them feels less like effort and more like a natural way of living.

Part 4
The 30-Day Liver Healing Plan

Chapter 12: Full Recipe Guide

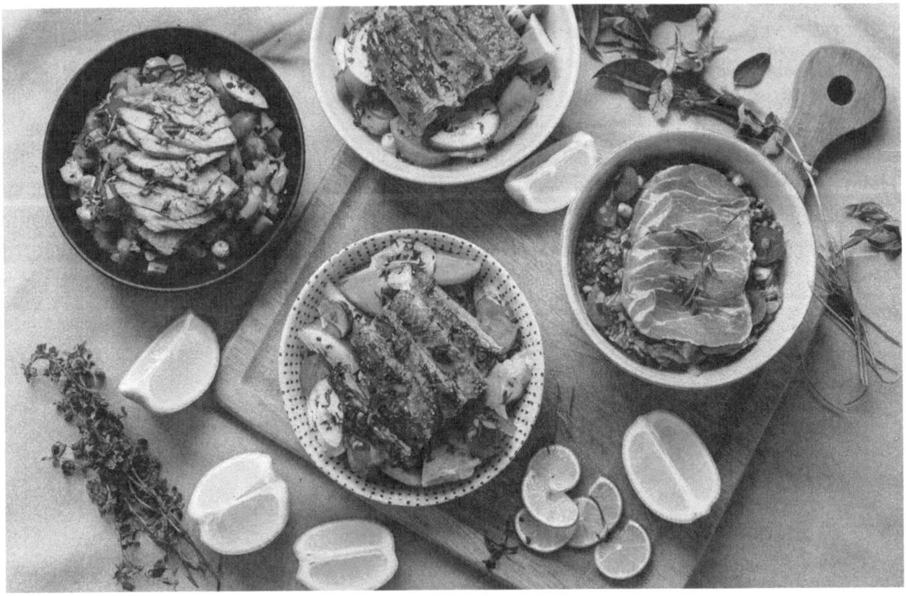

Breakfast Recipes for Liver Support

Breakfast is an opportunity to start the day with nutrient-rich, anti-inflammatory foods that provide steady energy while supporting digestion and liver regeneration. The goal is to combine fiber, protein, healthy fats, and phytonutrients in a way that is easy to digest and energizing.

Avocado and Spinach Smoothie

This creamy smoothie blends avocado for healthy fats, spinach for antioxidants and magnesium, and unsweetened almond milk for a light base. Add a tablespoon of ground flaxseed for extra fiber and omega-3s, and a handful of berries for natural sweetness. This combination supports bile flow, reduces inflammation, and provides lasting energy.

Turmeric Oatmeal

Steel-cut oats are cooked slowly in water or unsweetened almond milk until tender, then stirred with turmeric powder, cinnamon, and a small amount of black pepper to enhance curcumin absorption. Top with blueberries and a sprinkle of walnuts for antioxidants and healthy fats. This meal stabilizes blood sugar while delivering anti-inflammatory compounds.

Poached Eggs on Wilted Greens

Two eggs are poached and served over lightly sautéed kale or Swiss chard cooked in olive oil and garlic. A squeeze of lemon brightens the flavor and helps with iron absorption. The combination of high-quality protein, leafy greens, and healthy fats gives the liver the raw materials it needs for repair.

Chia and Flax Pudding with Berries

Chia seeds and ground flaxseed are soaked overnight in unsweetened oat milk. In the morning, top with fresh strawberries and a drizzle of raw honey. The soluble fiber supports healthy digestion and toxin elimination, while the omega-3s aid in reducing liver inflammation.

Apple and Cinnamon Quinoa Breakfast Bowl

Cooked quinoa is warmed with diced apples, cinnamon, and a splash of unsweetened coconut milk. A handful of pumpkin seeds adds crunch and zinc, an essential mineral for liver enzyme function.

Ginger and Pear Smoothie

Blend ripe pear with fresh ginger, spinach, unsweetened soy milk, and hemp seeds. Ginger aids digestion and circulation, while pear provides soluble fiber for gentle detox support.

Sweet Potato and Black Bean Hash

Diced sweet potatoes are roasted until tender, then tossed with black beans, chopped red peppers, and fresh cilantro. This meal is rich in beta-carotene, fiber, and plant-based protein, all of which support liver regeneration.

Lunch Recipes for Liver Health

Lunch should deliver a balance of macronutrients while remaining light enough to keep energy stable throughout the afternoon. Fiber-rich vegetables, lean proteins, and healthy fats are central here.

Grilled Salmon with Lemon Dill Quinoa

Salmon provides omega-3 fatty acids that help reduce liver fat and inflammation. Serve with fluffy quinoa tossed in lemon juice, fresh dill, and chopped parsley for a refreshing, anti-inflammatory side.

Lentil and Spinach Stew

Brown lentils are simmered with diced carrots, celery, onion, and vegetable broth until tender. A few handfuls of spinach are stirred in just before serving. Lentils provide plant-based protein and fiber, while spinach delivers folate and magnesium for metabolic support.

Mediterranean Chickpea Salad

Combine chickpeas, cucumber, tomatoes, red onion, parsley, and Kalamata olives with olive oil and lemon dressing. This salad is rich in antioxidants, healthy fats, and fiber, which together help stabilize blood sugar and reduce oxidative stress.

Zucchini Noodles with Basil Pesto

Fresh zucchini noodles are tossed with homemade pesto made from basil, olive oil, walnuts, garlic, and lemon juice. This grain-free option is light, anti-inflammatory, and rich in phytonutrients.

Roasted Beet and Arugula Salad

Roasted beets are sliced and layered over peppery arugula with crumbled goat cheese, toasted pumpkin seeds, and a light balsamic vinaigrette. Beets support bile flow and detoxification, while arugula adds vitamin K and antioxidants.

Miso and Vegetable Soup

A light broth made from miso paste and water is simmered with bok choy, shiitake mushrooms, carrots, and tofu. The fermented miso provides probiotics that support the gut–liver axis.

Stuffed Bell Peppers with Turkey and Brown Rice

Red and yellow bell peppers are filled with a mixture of lean ground turkey, cooked brown rice, onions, and herbs. This meal is high in protein, fiber, and antioxidants that protect liver cells.

Wholesome Dinners for Liver Repair

Dinner is the time to provide the body with nutrient-dense foods that assist overnight detoxification and liver regeneration. Evening meals should include moderate portions of lean protein, vegetables, and healthy fats.

Lemon Herb Chicken with Steamed Broccoli

Skinless chicken breast is marinated in lemon juice, garlic, and fresh thyme before baking until tender. Serve with steamed broccoli and a drizzle of olive oil. The citrus helps with iron absorption, while broccoli supports natural detox pathways.

Quinoa Stuffed Peppers

Large bell peppers are stuffed with quinoa, sautéed zucchini, onions, and fresh herbs, then baked until tender. This plant-focused dish offers fiber, plant protein, and anti-inflammatory nutrients.

Baked Cod with Tomato and Olive Tapenade

Cod fillets are topped with a mixture of chopped tomatoes, olives, capers, and parsley, then baked until flaky. This Mediterranean-inspired dish is light, flavorful, and rich in antioxidants.

Vegetable and Lentil Curry

A blend of carrots, cauliflower, zucchini, and lentils is simmered with turmeric, cumin, ginger, and coconut milk. This warm dish provides anti-inflammatory benefits along with fiber and plant-based protein.

Grilled Eggplant with Tahini Sauce

Thick slices of eggplant are grilled until soft, then drizzled with tahini, lemon juice, and fresh parsley. Eggplant offers antioxidants and fiber, while tahini delivers healthy fats and minerals like magnesium.

Wild Rice and Mushroom Pilaf with Baked Salmon

Wild rice is cooked with vegetable broth, onions, and sautéed mushrooms, then paired with oven-baked salmon. This combination provides slow-digesting carbohydrates, protein, and anti-inflammatory omega-3s.

Cauliflower Rice Stir-Fry with Shrimp

Cauliflower rice is sautéed with garlic, ginger, mixed vegetables, and shrimp for a light but satisfying dinner. This low-glycemic option supports stable blood sugar and reduces the liver's fat storage burden.

Meal Preparation and Practical Tips

The success of a 30-day liver healing plan depends on more than the recipes themselves. Planning and preparation can make it easier to stick to the fatty liver diet plan without feeling overwhelmed.

Batch cooking grains such as quinoa or brown rice early in the week allows you to use them in multiple recipes. Pre-washing and chopping vegetables makes it quicker to prepare salads, stir-fries, and side dishes. Keeping pantry staples like olive oil, nuts, seeds, and herbs on hand ensures you always have the building blocks of liver-friendly meals.

Portion control is another key element. Meals that are too large, even when made from healthy ingredients, can slow digestion and tax the liver. Eating until comfortably satisfied, rather than full, helps maintain energy balance and supports digestion.

Hydration should also be integrated with meals. While drinking small amounts of water during eating is fine, larger amounts are best consumed between meals to avoid diluting digestive enzymes.

For variety and to maintain motivation, rotate proteins and vegetables each week. Try swapping salmon for trout, quinoa for millet, or kale for bok choy. This variety not only prevents boredom but also ensures you are getting a wide spectrum of nutrients.

Healthy Liver-Friendly Snacks

Snacks can either work for your liver or against it. For those following a fatty liver diet plan, snacks should support stable blood sugar, improve digestion naturally, and provide nutrients that promote liver regeneration. They should be easy to prepare, portable if needed, and satisfying without excess sugar or processed ingredients. A smart snack can bridge the gap between meals without overburdening the liver.

Almond Energy Bites

These small, nutrient-dense bites are made from almonds, dates, chia seeds, and unsweetened cocoa powder. The almonds supply vitamin E, a powerful antioxidant that helps reduce liver inflammation, while chia seeds provide omega-3s and fiber. Dates give natural sweetness without refined sugar, and cocoa offers polyphenols that benefit circulation. The ingredients are blended, rolled into small balls, and stored in the refrigerator for quick access.

Cucumber Roll-Ups

Thinly sliced cucumber is spread with hummus and wrapped around thin strips of bell pepper or carrot. This refreshing snack is high in antioxidants and fiber while being gentle on digestion. The cucumbers provide hydration, and the hummus delivers plant protein and healthy fats from olive oil and tahini.

Pumpkin Seed and Berry Mix

A simple mix of raw pumpkin seeds, freeze-dried blueberries, and unsweetened coconut flakes makes a portable snack rich in magnesium, antioxidants, and healthy fats. Pumpkin seeds support liver enzyme function, while blueberries help reduce oxidative stress.

Roasted Chickpeas with Turmeric

Chickpeas are tossed with olive oil, turmeric, and a pinch of black pepper, then roasted until crisp. This combination delivers plant-based protein, anti-inflammatory benefits, and a satisfying crunch without refined carbohydrates.

Apple Slices with Walnut Butter

Crisp apple slices are paired with walnut butter, providing soluble fiber for digestive health and omega-3s to help reverse fatty liver. The natural sweetness of the apple complements the richness of the walnuts.

Some snacks in a liver health guide are more than just “filler” between meals. When designed with nutrients in mind, they can act as small doses of targeted therapy, helping to maintain energy, balance hormones, and keep the liver’s detox pathways moving efficiently.

Herbal Teas for Liver Health

Herbal teas are a gentle yet powerful way to support liver function. They can be sipped throughout the day, delivering beneficial compounds that help reduce liver inflammation, promote bile flow, and protect liver cells from oxidative stress. For those working to reverse fatty liver, herbal teas fit easily into an anti-inflammatory diet.

Milk Thistle Tea

Milk thistle contains silymarin, known for its antioxidant and liver-regenerating properties. When consumed as tea, it provides a soothing, caffeine-free way to deliver this compound. It is often combined with other herbs such as peppermint or ginger for improved flavor and additional digestive support.

Turmeric-Fennel Tea

Turmeric reduces inflammation and supports bile production, while fennel helps ease bloating and improve digestion naturally. This tea can be made by simmering fresh turmeric root with fennel seeds, then straining and adding a squeeze of lemon for vitamin C.

Dandelion Root Tea

Dandelion root stimulates bile flow, supports detoxification, and may help lower liver enzyme levels in people with mild liver stress. It has a slightly earthy flavor that can be balanced with cinnamon or ginger.

Ginger and Lemon Balm Tea

Ginger aids circulation and digestion, while lemon balm provides mild calming effects that help lower stress-related inflammation. This combination supports both the gut–liver axis and overall energy.

Green Tea with Mint

Green tea contains catechins, which have been studied for their potential to reduce liver fat and improve enzyme profiles. Adding mint makes the tea more refreshing and may soothe digestion after meals.

Herbal teas are not just beverages in a fatty liver diet plan. These functional remedies can be tailored to specific needs. For example, dandelion root tea might be favored during a focused detox phase, while ginger and lemon balm could be chosen during times of stress.

Smoothies for Liver Health

Smoothies can be an effective way to deliver concentrated nutrients in an easy-to-digest form. They work especially well in a liver health guide because they allow for combinations of anti-inflammatory fruits, leafy greens, healthy fats, and herbs that promote liver regeneration. The key is to avoid adding excessive sugar and instead focus on ingredients that help reverse fatty liver.

Berry Detox Smoothie

Berries are among the best fruits for reducing oxidative stress and supporting an anti-inflammatory diet. In this smoothie, blueberries, blackberries, and raspberries are blended with unsweetened almond milk, spinach, and ground flaxseed. The combination provides antioxidants, fiber, and plant-based omega-3s. A small amount of fresh ginger adds a gentle digestive boost.

Pineapple Turmeric Smoothie

Fresh pineapple contains bromelain, an enzyme that supports protein digestion, while turmeric provides curcumin for inflammation control. Blending these with coconut water, a banana, and a spoonful of chia seeds creates a refreshing, hydrating option that also supports bile flow.

Avocado and Kale Smoothie

This smoothie combines avocado for healthy fats and creaminess with kale for vitamins A, C, and K, all essential for liver repair. Adding a small green apple and cucumber balances the flavor and provides hydration. A squeeze of lemon brightens the taste and helps with iron absorption from the kale.

Beet and Carrot Liver Cleanser

Beets support bile flow and detoxification, while carrots provide beta-carotene for cell repair. Blending them with orange segments, ginger, and a little water produces a naturally sweet drink packed with liver-friendly compounds.

Papaya Mint Smoothie

Papaya contains enzymes that aid digestion, while mint adds freshness and supports the gut–liver connection. Blended with coconut milk and a handful of spinach, this smoothie delivers fiber, antioxidants, and healthy fats in a gentle, soothing package.

Practical Tips for Snack, Tea, and Smoothie Integration

To make these snacks, teas, and smoothies work seamlessly in a fatty liver diet plan, preparation and timing are key. Snacks should be portioned in advance to avoid overeating, even with healthy ingredients. Herbal teas can be brewed in larger batches and stored in the refrigerator for iced versions, making them easy to sip throughout the day.

Smoothies are best consumed fresh to preserve antioxidants, although they can be stored for a few hours in an insulated container if needed. Balancing smoothie ingredients with adequate protein and healthy fat helps maintain stable energy and prevent sugar spikes, even when using naturally sweet fruits.

Rather than just being additions to the 30-day liver healing plan, these are tools for building daily habits that support liver regeneration, reduce inflammation, and maintain results for the long term.

Chapter 13: Week 1 — Detox Kickstart

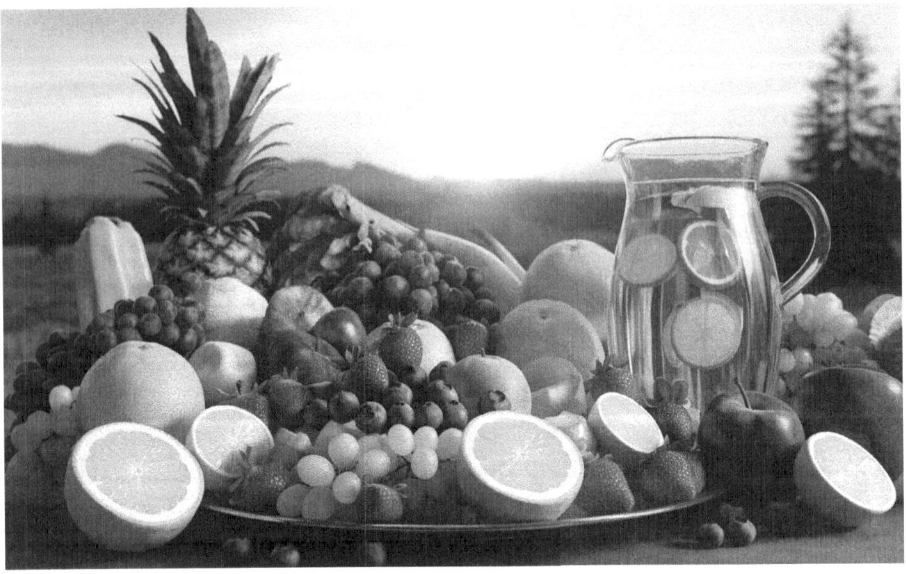

1. Remove Harmful Foods and Environmental Toxins

The first step in a liver regeneration program is to stop the constant influx of substances that damage liver cells and slow healing. Many people focus only on food changes, but environmental toxins also contribute to liver inflammation and fatty liver progression.

From a dietary perspective, processed foods with high amounts of refined sugar, trans fats, and additives should be eliminated right away. This includes sodas, packaged snacks, pastries, fried fast food, and heavily processed meats. These foods cause blood sugar spikes, increase triglycerides, and create oxidative stress, all of which overload detox pathways.

In addition to dietary changes, removing common environmental toxins from daily life can make a big difference. Switching to natural cleaning products reduces exposure to volatile compounds that the liver must process. Storing food in glass or stainless steel instead of plastic lowers contact with chemicals like BPA. Choosing organic produce for high-pesticide items further reduces toxic load.

The idea is to create an environment, internally and externally, where the liver is no longer fighting constant new damage, freeing its resources for repair and regeneration.

2. Establish a Liver-Healing Hydration Routine

Hydration is more than just drinking water when you feel thirsty. For optimal liver regeneration, water intake should be steady and spread throughout the day to maintain circulation and nutrient transport.

Starting the day with a glass of warm water infused with lemon helps stimulate bile flow and kickstart digestion. From there, aim for small, frequent sips of water rather than consuming large amounts all at once. This prevents overloading the kidneys and allows better hydration of tissues.

While plain water is best, herbal teas that reduce liver inflammation or improve digestion can be included. Dandelion tea, ginger tea, and green tea are all excellent choices for supporting detox processes in week one. Coconut water can be used occasionally for electrolytes, but avoid those with added sugar.

It is important to reduce beverages that slow progress, such as alcohol, sugary drinks, and excessive coffee. While a moderate amount of black coffee can have antioxidant benefits, too much caffeine increases stress hormones and may interfere with sleep, which is crucial for liver repair.

3. Implement Sleep and Recovery Protocols

Sleep is one of the most underestimated factors in a liver health guide. The liver performs much of its regeneration and detoxification during deep sleep. Without sufficient rest, even the best fatty liver diet plan will have slower results.

During week one, the goal is to create a consistent sleep schedule. Going to bed and waking up at the same time each day helps regulate the body's circadian rhythm, which in turn supports liver function. Ideally, aim for seven to nine hours of quality sleep.

Reducing screen time before bed, keeping the bedroom cool and dark, and avoiding large meals or caffeine in the evening all help improve sleep quality. Light stretching or breathing exercises before bed can further prepare the body for restful sleep. Recovery also involves minimizing excessive physical stress during the first week, as the body is adapting to dietary changes and increased detox activity.

4. Gentle Gallbladder and Liver Cleanse Practices

The liver and gallbladder work closely together. The liver produces bile, which is stored and concentrated in the gallbladder before being released into the digestive tract to help break down fats and remove fat-soluble toxins. In week one, the goal is to encourage gentle bile flow rather than aggressive cleanses that may overwhelm the system.

Incorporating bitter greens like arugula, dandelion leaves, and endive into meals can stimulate bile production naturally. Beets and artichokes are particularly supportive for both the liver and gallbladder. Healthy fats in moderate amounts, such as avocado, olive oil, and walnuts, also encourage bile release without straining digestion.

A simple morning ritual to support bile flow is to drink warm water with lemon before eating breakfast. This primes the digestive system and sets the tone for improved fat metabolism throughout the day.

5. Herbal Support for Initial Detox

Herbs can play a gentle but important role in the first week of a detox-focused fatty liver diet plan. They can help reduce liver inflammation, improve circulation, and support the detox pathways without causing sudden or extreme reactions.

Milk thistle is one of the best-known natural remedies for liver health. Its active compound, silymarin, helps protect liver cells and supports regeneration. Dandelion root is another excellent choice, as it aids digestion and promotes bile flow. Turmeric, with its anti-inflammatory compound curcumin, can be added to meals or consumed as a tea for additional support.

Other gentle herbs for week one include peppermint for digestive comfort, ginger for circulation and digestive stimulation, and burdock root for blood purification. These can be rotated throughout the week in teas or incorporated into cooking.

6. Week 1 Meal Plan and Recipes

The week one meal plan focuses on reducing inflammatory load, improving nutrient density, and supporting digestion without overwhelming the system. Meals are balanced to maintain stable blood sugar and provide the vitamins and minerals needed for liver regeneration.

Breakfast Options

- Avocado and spinach smoothie made with unsweetened almond milk, chia seeds, and a handful of blueberries
- Turmeric oatmeal with ground flaxseed, cinnamon, and sliced pear
- Poached eggs served over sautéed kale and mushrooms with a squeeze of lemon

Lunch Options

- Lentil and vegetable soup with carrots, celery, and garlic, served with a side of mixed greens
- Grilled salmon with steamed broccoli and lemon-dill quinoa
- Mediterranean chickpea salad with cucumber, tomato, red onion, parsley, and olive oil

Dinner Options

- Baked cod with roasted beets and arugula salad
- Vegetable curry with cauliflower, zucchini, spinach, and chickpeas in a coconut milk base
- Quinoa-stuffed bell peppers with zucchini, onions, and fresh herbs

Snack Ideas

- Apple slices with walnut butter

- Cucumber roll-ups with hummus and carrot sticks
- A small handful of raw pumpkin seeds with a few dried goji berries

Example Day in Week One

Morning:

Start with warm lemon water, followed by a breakfast of turmeric oatmeal with flaxseed and pear.

Midday:

Sip on dandelion root tea and have a Mediterranean chickpea salad for lunch.

Afternoon Snack:

Enjoy cucumber roll-ups and a handful of pumpkin seeds.

Evening:

Have baked cod with roasted beets and arugula salad, followed by ginger tea to aid digestion before bed.

This structure ensures each day provides steady energy, keeps digestion light, and focuses on whole, anti-inflammatory foods. By the end of week one, many people notice reduced bloating, improved digestion, and a gentle lift in energy as the liver begins to function more efficiently.

Chapter 14: Week 2
Deep Detox and Gut Health

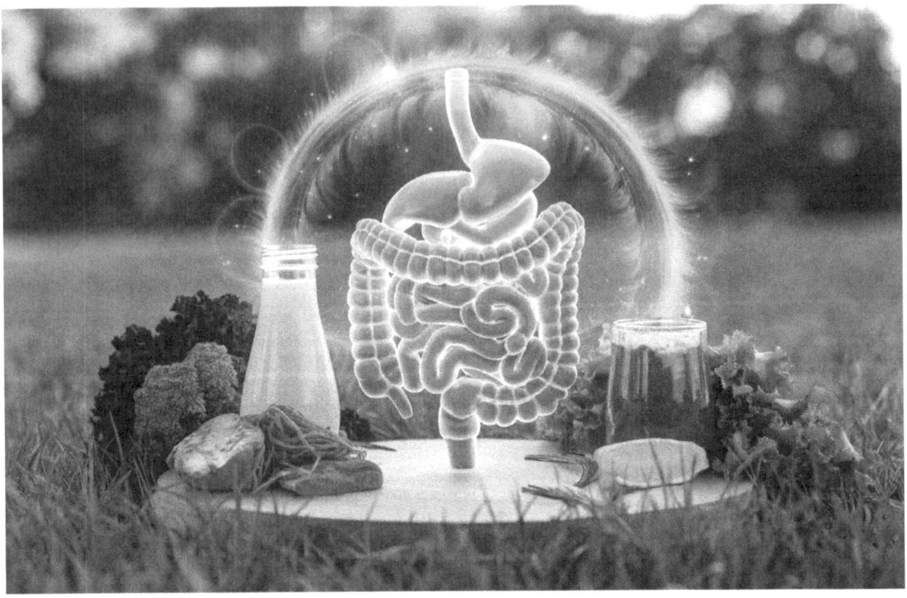

1. Start the Liver Detox Diet and Nutrient Loading

Week two builds on the foundation of week one by introducing a more targeted liver detox diet that focuses on nutrient loading. This means flooding the body with vitamins, minerals, antioxidants, and phytonutrients that the liver needs for repair and regeneration while still maintaining a gentle approach to detoxification. The goal is not to starve the body but to feed it with the raw materials needed for deep cellular recovery.

During this week, meals should become more plant-forward while still including adequate protein to support detox enzymes. More cruciferous vegetables such as broccoli, cauliflower, and Brussels sprouts are added because they contain compounds that activate phase two detoxification in the liver. Leafy greens like kale, collard greens, and arugula help maintain alkaline balance and promote healthy bile flow.

Nutrient-dense fruits such as blueberries, pomegranate seeds, and kiwi are included for their high antioxidant content. Whole grains like quinoa and millet are preferred over refined carbohydrates to stabilize blood sugar and avoid adding fat to the liver. Healthy fats from olive oil, walnuts, and chia seeds are used daily to reduce inflammation and aid in the absorption of fat-soluble vitamins.

Reducing sodium while increasing herbs and spices is also important this week. Turmeric, rosemary, oregano, and cinnamon help reduce liver inflammation naturally while adding flavor without processed sauces or additives.

2. Gut–Liver Axis Support for Regeneration

The gut–liver axis is a bidirectional communication pathway between the digestive tract and the liver. What happens in the gut affects the liver, and vice versa. In week two, special focus is placed on improving gut integrity so fewer toxins and inflammatory compounds reach the liver through the portal vein.

Supporting gut health starts with increasing prebiotic and probiotic foods. Prebiotics are fibers that feed beneficial gut bacteria. They are found in foods like garlic, onions, leeks, asparagus, and artichokes. Probiotics are live bacteria found in fermented foods such as sauerkraut, kimchi, kefir, and unsweetened yogurt. Together, these foods help restore microbiome balance and reduce endotoxin leakage into the bloodstream.

Digestive enzymes are also encouraged in week two, either from supplemental sources or naturally occurring in foods like pineapple (bromelain) and papaya (papain). These enzymes improve nutrient absorption, which supports liver regeneration.

This week, it is also recommended to avoid inflammatory gut irritants such as excessive caffeine, alcohol, and ultra-processed snacks. Even small amounts of alcohol can slow liver repair during a detox phase. The less strain placed on digestion, the more energy the liver can devote to healing.

3. Introduce Intermittent Fasting for Liver Health

Intermittent fasting is introduced this week as a gentle metabolic reset tool. The most beginner-friendly approach is the 12:12 method, eating within a 12-hour window and fasting for the other 12. As the body adapts, the eating window can be reduced to 10 hours or even 8 hours if energy levels remain stable.

Fasting periods give the liver a break from constant nutrient processing, allowing it to focus on detoxification and fat metabolism. During the fasting window, the body begins to mobilize stored fat for energy, which can help reverse fatty liver over time. Fasting also improves insulin sensitivity, reducing the risk of additional fat accumulation in the liver.

It is important that meals within the eating window are nutrient-dense and balanced. This prevents blood sugar crashes and ensures that the liver receives the vitamins and minerals needed for regeneration. Fasting is not about eating less food overall, but rather about timing meals to work with the body's natural repair cycles.

4. Supplements for Liver and Gut Repair

Week two is also the time to introduce supplements that support both the liver and the gut. These are not a replacement for whole foods but can enhance recovery.

Milk thistle extract provides silymarin, which helps repair liver cells and protects them from oxidative stress. NAC (N-acetyl cysteine) boosts glutathione production, which is essential for detoxification. Turmeric or curcumin supplements can be used for additional anti-inflammatory support, ideally taken with black pepper extract to improve absorption.

For gut repair, a high-quality probiotic supplement can help restore microbiome diversity, especially if fermented foods are not consumed daily. L-glutamine powder may be used to help strengthen the intestinal lining, preventing harmful compounds from leaking into the bloodstream and overburdening the liver. Digestive enzyme supplements can also improve nutrient absorption and reduce bloating.

These supplements should be introduced gradually to observe how the body responds. Overloading on too many new products at once can make it difficult to identify what is helping and what may be causing discomfort.

5. Week 2 Meal Plan and Recipes

The week two meal plan continues to follow an anti-inflammatory diet but increases the volume of raw and lightly cooked vegetables, fermented foods, and antioxidant-rich fruits. Protein remains steady to preserve muscle mass and support detox enzymes.

Breakfast Options

- Blueberry and spinach smoothie with chia seeds, unsweetened almond milk, and a teaspoon of flaxseed oil for omega-3s
- Scrambled eggs with sautéed mushrooms, garlic, and kale, served with a side of fermented sauerkraut
- Quinoa breakfast bowl with sliced kiwi, hemp seeds, cinnamon, and a drizzle of almond butter

Lunch Options

- Mediterranean quinoa salad with cucumbers, tomatoes, parsley, lemon juice, olive oil, and grilled salmon
- Lentil and vegetable soup with garlic, leeks, carrots, and celery, served with a side of steamed broccoli
- Zucchini noodles tossed with basil pesto made from walnuts, olive oil, fresh basil, and garlic

Dinner Options

- Baked cod with roasted asparagus, beetroot, and a side of wild rice
- Chickpea and vegetable curry with cauliflower, zucchini, and spinach in a light coconut milk sauce
- Turkey and spinach lettuce wraps with avocado, shredded carrots, and sesame seeds

Snack Ideas

- A small bowl of unsweetened yogurt with pomegranate seeds and pumpkin seeds
- Sliced cucumber and celery with hummus made from garlic, lemon juice, and tahini
- A handful of raw walnuts with fresh raspberries

Example Day in Week Two

Morning:

Begin with a glass of warm lemon water, followed by a blueberry and spinach smoothie with chia seeds and flaxseed oil.

Midday:

Enjoy Mediterranean quinoa salad with cucumbers, tomatoes, lemon juice, olive oil, parsley, and grilled salmon.

Afternoon Snack:

Have cucumber and celery sticks with homemade hummus.

Evening:

Baked cod with roasted asparagus and beets, served alongside wild rice, followed by ginger tea for digestion.

This daily structure not only supports liver regeneration but also provides ongoing gut–liver axis support through high fiber intake, probiotics, and anti-inflammatory foods.

Chapter 15: Week 3
Energy Boost and Metabolism Reset

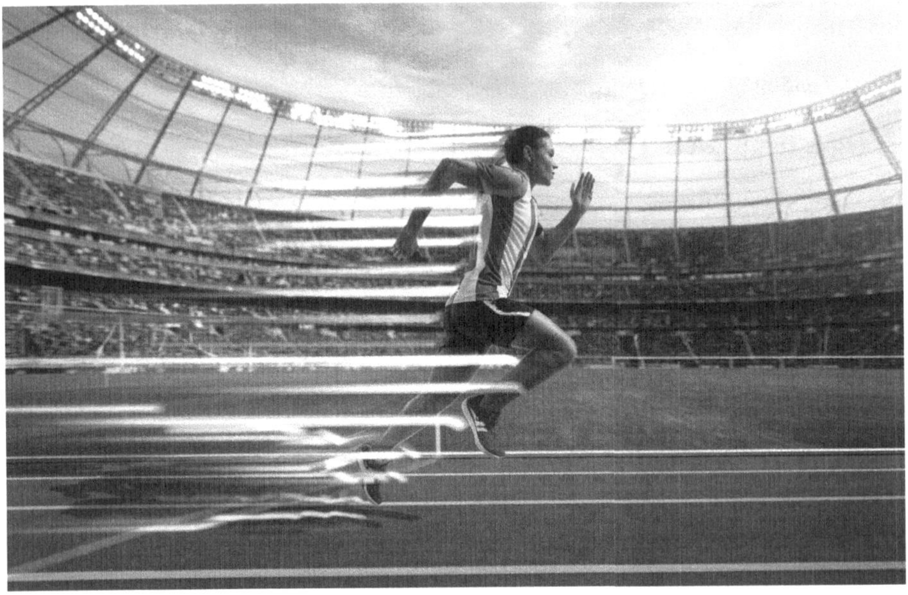

1. Add Liver-Healing Superfoods to Daily Routine

Week three focuses on introducing nutrient-dense superfoods that help the liver work more efficiently, reduce inflammation, and provide sustained energy. These foods are not exotic gimmicks but whole, natural ingredients supported by research for their role in liver regeneration.

Leafy greens such as kale, collard greens, and spinach are priority items this week because they help increase bile production and provide chlorophyll, which supports detoxification. Cruciferous vegetables like broccoli and Brussels sprouts contain compounds that assist the liver's phase two detox pathways, improving its ability to remove harmful compounds from the body.

Beets are another valuable addition because they help support blood flow and bile production. Including small amounts of beet in salads, juices, or roasted dishes can be an easy habit to maintain. Garlic and onions provide sulfur compounds that help neutralize toxins and reduce oxidative stress inside liver cells.

Antioxidant-rich fruits such as blueberries, blackberries, and pomegranate seeds are introduced more frequently this week. They help reduce liver inflammation and improve blood flow, both of which are important for reversing fatty liver. Turmeric, preferably paired with black pepper for better absorption, is used in cooking or added to herbal teas for anti-inflammatory benefits.

Healthy fats from walnuts, chia seeds, and flaxseeds provide omega-3 fatty acids that help regulate triglyceride levels and improve metabolic balance. These foods also keep energy stable by slowing glucose release into the bloodstream.

2. Adjust Exercise and Movement for Liver Support

Physical activity in week three moves beyond gentle detox support and begins targeting metabolism improvement. The aim is to encourage the body to use stored fat for energy, helping to reverse fatty liver and improve insulin sensitivity.

If you have been walking daily in previous weeks, now is the time to add short bursts of moderate-intensity activity. This could include brisk walking, cycling, swimming, or bodyweight exercises such as squats and lunges. These movements improve circulation, allowing nutrients to reach liver cells more effectively while carrying away waste products.

Strength training is particularly valuable at this stage because muscle tissue is metabolically active. Even two short sessions per week using resistance bands or light weights can increase resting metabolic rate, which supports the metabolic reset program. Improved muscle mass also makes it easier to maintain stable blood sugar, which reduces the risk of fat being stored in the liver.

Movement should still be balanced with recovery. Overtraining or suddenly engaging in intense exercise can trigger fatigue and slow liver healing. It is better to make gradual adjustments, listening to how the body responds and increasing activity at a sustainable pace.

3. Managing Detox Symptoms and Energy Fluctuations

By week three, the body is processing and eliminating stored toxins more efficiently, but this can lead to temporary discomfort if the detox pace is faster than the body can eliminate waste. Common symptoms include mild headaches, changes in digestion, or temporary dips in energy.

Managing these symptoms begins with hydration. Drinking water steadily throughout the day helps flush toxins through the kidneys and prevent them from being reabsorbed. Adding lemon or cucumber slices can make hydration more appealing while supporting digestion.

Adequate fiber intake is also critical for binding toxins in the digestive tract and moving them out of the body. This means continuing to include vegetables, fruits, legumes, and whole grains in every meal. Fermented foods like sauerkraut or kefir help maintain gut health during detox and keep digestion regular.

If energy levels dip, small adjustments such as adding a mid-morning snack of berries and walnuts or a small smoothie with spinach and chia seeds can provide a nutrient boost without overloading digestion. Gentle stretching, walking, or deep breathing can help improve circulation and relieve mild detox-related fatigue.

It is also important to avoid unnecessary environmental toxin exposure at this stage. Reducing synthetic fragrances, harsh cleaning products, and pesticide-heavy produce can keep the detox load manageable.

4. Metabolic Boost Strategies for Fatty Liver Reversal

Reversing fatty liver and restoring metabolic balance requires addressing how the body stores and uses energy. In week three, the focus shifts to supporting mitochondria, the energy powerhouses in cells, and optimizing fuel use.

One strategy is to maintain balanced macronutrient intake at each meal. Including lean proteins, healthy fats, and complex carbohydrates helps prevent spikes and crashes in blood sugar, which can otherwise contribute to fat buildup in the liver.

Incorporating thermogenic spices like cinnamon, cayenne, and ginger into meals can give a mild metabolic lift while also supporting digestion. These can be added to smoothies, soups, or roasted vegetables.

Keeping evening meals lighter can also help the metabolic reset program. The liver is more efficient at processing nutrients earlier in the day, so having heavier meals in the morning or early afternoon can improve fat metabolism and leave more energy available for overnight repair.

Daily activity remains a key metabolic booster. Even on rest days, incorporating movement such as gentle yoga, stretching, or light housework can keep circulation active and prevent energy stagnation.

5. Week 3 Meal Plan and Recipes

Week three meals emphasize superfoods for liver regeneration, anti-inflammatory ingredients, and balanced portions to keep metabolism efficient.

Breakfast Options

- Spinach and mushroom omelet cooked in olive oil, served with a side of blueberries
- Chia seed pudding made with unsweetened almond milk, topped with pomegranate seeds and walnuts
- Turmeric-spiced quinoa porridge with cinnamon, pear slices, and pumpkin seeds

Lunch Options

- Grilled chicken salad with mixed greens, roasted beets, avocado, and lemon-tahini dressing
- Lentil and vegetable stew with garlic, carrots, celery, and fresh parsley
- Quinoa and chickpea bowl with steamed broccoli, shredded carrots, and ginger dressing

Dinner Options

- Baked salmon with Brussels sprouts, sweet potato mash, and a sprinkle of fresh dill
- Vegetable stir-fry with bok choy, bell peppers, and shiitake mushrooms served over wild rice
- Roasted cauliflower steaks topped with turmeric sauce, served with a side of arugula and cucumber salad

Snack Ideas

- Cucumber slices with hummus
- A handful of almonds with fresh raspberries
- Apple slices with chia-almond butter spread

Example Day in Week Three

Morning:

Start with warm lemon water followed by a spinach and mushroom omelet with blueberries on the side.

Midday:

Have a quinoa and chickpea bowl with steamed broccoli, shredded carrots, and ginger dressing.

Afternoon Snack:

Enjoy cucumber slices with hummus.

Evening:

Baked salmon with Brussels sprouts, sweet potato mash, and fresh dill, followed by a cup of ginger tea to support digestion before bed.

This week's plan blends the nutrient density needed for liver healing with the balanced energy sources necessary for metabolism reset. By the end of week three, many people notice greater stamina, improved digestion, and a more stable energy pattern throughout the day.

Chapter 16: Week 4
Long-Term Liver Optimization

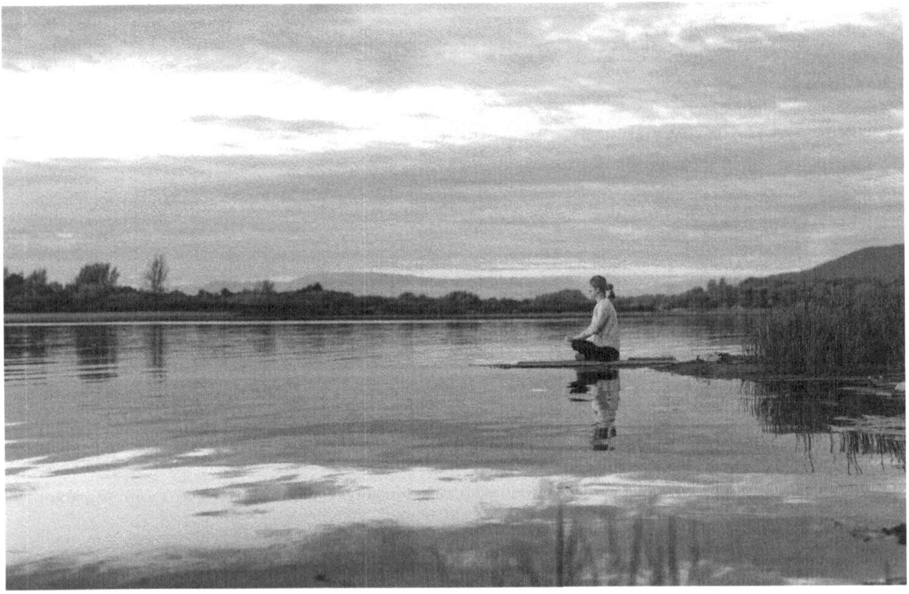

1. Maintain Liver Health Habits Long-Term

By week four, the liver has already benefited from a consistent anti-inflammatory diet, targeted nutrients, and reduced exposure to harmful substances. Now the focus shifts to creating a lifestyle that keeps these gains for the long term. Short-term improvements are encouraging, but lasting liver regeneration requires ongoing habits that become second nature.

This means continuing to choose whole foods over processed ones, cooking at home more often, and keeping hydration a daily priority. It also means maintaining regular physical activity and setting aside time for restorative sleep. The body thrives on consistency, and the liver in particular benefits from a steady flow of nutrients rather than a pattern of intense health focus followed by neglect.

Meal planning is an important part of maintaining these habits. It prevents last-minute food choices that could derail progress and ensures your kitchen remains stocked with liver-friendly staples. Weekly shopping lists can be built around core items such as leafy greens, cruciferous vegetables, high-quality proteins, and healthy fats. Even when life gets busy, these habits form a safety net for liver health.

2. Reintroduce Foods and Maintain Balance

After several weeks of following a clean and highly structured fatty liver diet plan, some foods that were reduced or removed can be reintroduced in moderation. The goal is to expand food variety without triggering inflammation or fat buildup in the liver.

Start with foods that are minimally processed and nutrient-rich, even if they were limited earlier. For example, small amounts of whole-grain bread or sprouted grain products may be reintroduced if they are well tolerated. Starchy vegetables such as sweet corn or potatoes can return in modest portions alongside fiber-rich greens.

Portion control is essential during this phase. Reintroduction is not an invitation to return to old eating patterns but rather a way to diversify nutrients while monitoring how the body responds. Keeping a simple food journal can help identify any digestive discomfort, energy dips, or changes in mood that follow certain foods.

Some items, like refined sugars, deep-fried foods, and high-sodium processed snacks, are best avoided long-term. Even occasional indulgences should be balanced with nutrient-rich meals before and after to reduce the impact on the liver. This balance is key for sustainable results and helps ensure that small dietary changes do not lead to gradual relapse.

3. Track Liver Enzyme Levels and Progress

Laboratory testing is one of the most reliable ways to confirm that the liver health improvements you feel are also occurring at a biological level. Blood tests for ALT, AST, GGT, and ALP provide measurable indicators of liver function. Bilirubin and albumin levels can also give insight into the liver's ability to process waste and produce essential proteins.

Testing every three to six months during the first year of a lifestyle change allows you to track progress and make adjustments as needed. If enzyme levels remain elevated, it may indicate that inflammation is still present or that dietary and lifestyle changes need fine-tuning. In some cases, additional testing such as ultrasound or FibroScan may be recommended to assess fat content or fibrosis.

Keeping your own record of results, alongside notes about diet, exercise, and stress levels, helps create a personalized liver health guide. Over time, patterns become clear, and you can see which changes have the most significant effect on your numbers.

4. Preventing Relapse and Cirrhosis

Preventing relapse is about maintaining both awareness and action. Once symptoms improve and enzyme levels normalize, it is easy to relax dietary and lifestyle habits. However, fatty liver can return if the factors that caused it are not managed long-term. This is particularly important because repeated cycles of damage and repair can increase the risk of fibrosis and cirrhosis.

Relapse prevention starts with keeping the primary triggers, poor diet, inactivity, excessive alcohol, unmanaged stress, under control. Alcohol, even in small amounts, can reverse progress for some individuals, especially if there is a history of inflammation or fibrosis. Monitoring weight and waist circumference can also help detect early signs of fat accumulation.

Stress management plays a bigger role than many people realize. Chronic stress influences hormone balance, blood sugar regulation, and inflammation, all of which affect liver health. Practices such as deep breathing, stretching, walking outdoors, or meditation are not just for relaxation. They help keep the liver's workload manageable.

Cirrhosis prevention goes beyond managing fatty liver. It includes vaccinations against hepatitis A and B, regular medical check-ups, and minimizing exposure to environmental toxins. Protecting the liver from further injury is crucial, especially for those who have already experienced moderate or advanced liver damage.

5. Week 4 Meal Plan and Recipes

Week four meals are designed for both nourishment and sustainability. They include enough variety to keep eating enjoyable while still following the principles of an anti-inflammatory diet.

Breakfast Options

- **Spinach and Avocado Omelet**: Two eggs with spinach, avocado slices, and fresh parsley cooked in olive oil.
- **Berry and Chia Pudding**: Chia seeds soaked overnight in unsweetened almond milk, topped with blueberries and pomegranate seeds.
- **Quinoa and Apple Breakfast Bowl**: Cooked quinoa with diced apple, cinnamon, pumpkin seeds, and a drizzle of almond butter.

Lunch Options

- **Mediterranean Lentil Salad**: Lentils, cucumber, tomato, red onion, parsley, olive oil, and lemon juice.
- **Salmon and Roasted Vegetables**: Baked salmon with roasted Brussels sprouts and carrots, seasoned with rosemary.
- **Chickpea and Spinach Soup**: Chickpeas simmered with garlic, spinach, celery, and vegetable broth.

Dinner Options

- **Lemon Herb Chicken with Wild Rice**: Chicken breast marinated in lemon juice, garlic, and thyme, served with wild rice and steamed broccoli.
- **Vegetable Stir-Fry with Tofu**: Mixed vegetables and tofu cooked with ginger, garlic, and a splash of low-sodium tamari, served over brown rice.
- **Baked Cod with Beet Salad**: Cod with roasted beets, arugula, walnuts, and balsamic vinaigrette.

Snack Ideas

- Handful of raw almonds and fresh raspberries.

- Sliced cucumber with hummus.
- Small bowl of unsweetened yogurt with flaxseed and kiwi.

Example Day in Week Four

Morning:

Start with warm lemon water. Breakfast is a spinach and avocado omelet with fresh parsley.

Midday:

Lunch is a Mediterranean lentil salad with olive oil and lemon juice.

Afternoon Snack:

Cucumber slices with hummus.

Evening:

Dinner is baked cod served with beet salad, arugula, walnuts, and balsamic vinaigrette, followed by a calming cup of chamomile tea.

This plan blends the nutrient density required for liver regeneration with the flexibility needed for long-term adherence. By week four, these recipes and habits should feel less like a "program" and more like a sustainable way of eating that supports energy, digestion, and ongoing liver health.

Conclusion: Sustaining Liver Health for Lifelong Vitality

The liver's ability to heal and regenerate is one of the body's most powerful tools for recovery, but long-term vitality depends on maintaining the habits that allowed it to improve in the first place. The journey to reverse fatty liver or reduce liver inflammation does not stop when enzyme levels normalize or when energy returns. Those milestones are the beginning of a lifelong commitment to protecting the liver and supporting its function every day.

Sustaining liver health means keeping a steady balance between nutrient intake, physical activity, and stress management. An anti-inflammatory diet rich in vegetables, lean proteins, healthy fats, and antioxidant-rich fruits forms the foundation. Hydration remains a daily priority, not just during structured programs. Consistent movement, whether through walking, strength training, or low-impact exercise, ensures circulation stays strong and the liver receives the oxygen and nutrients it needs.

Liver regeneration is not a one-time event but an ongoing process. Even when symptoms disappear, the liver continues to process toxins, regulate metabolism, and store essential nutrients. These processes work best in a supportive environment where harmful substances are minimized, nutrient levels are high, and inflammation is kept under control.

Moving Forward — Making the Changes Permanent

Permanent change happens when health habits feel like part of everyday life rather than short-term rules. A fatty liver diet plan works best when it is adaptable to different situations, from busy workweeks to family gatherings and holidays. That flexibility is what prevents old patterns from returning.

Meal planning remains an essential tool, but it can shift from a strict structure to a more intuitive approach as you learn which foods make you feel your best. The core principles — whole, minimally processed foods, balanced macronutrients, and mindful portions — stay the same, but there is room to experiment with flavors and recipes. This keeps meals interesting and makes it easier to sustain an anti-inflammatory diet long-term.

Small indulgences can fit into a healthy lifestyle as long as they are balanced with nutrient-rich choices. If a special occasion includes a dessert or richer meal, following it with lighter, vegetable-focused meals helps keep liver stress low. Awareness and moderation are more effective than rigid restriction for most people.

Continuing to monitor liver health through periodic check-ups ensures that progress is maintained. Tracking markers like ALT, AST, and GGT alongside energy levels, digestion, and mood provides a full picture of health. If any sign of relapse appears, adjustments can be made quickly before the liver is significantly affected.

Stress management also plays a central role in keeping results permanent. Chronic stress can disrupt blood sugar regulation, promote fat storage, and increase inflammation, all of which challenge liver health. Simple practices such as stretching, breathing exercises, or spending time outdoors can help maintain balance.

Building a Support Network for Ongoing Wellness

Health goals are easier to maintain with the right support. A personal network of friends, family, or community groups who understand and encourage liver-friendly habits can make a significant difference in long-term success. This support can come in many forms — from sharing healthy recipes to joining group walks or simply having someone to talk to about challenges and successes.

Working with healthcare professionals who understand both conventional medicine and natural remedies for liver health provides an additional layer of guidance. Nutritionists, functional medicine practitioners, or health coaches can help refine the fatty liver diet plan as your needs change over time. They can also recommend safe supplements or targeted nutrients when necessary, ensuring that these choices fit within your overall liver health guide.

For some, connecting with others who have reversed fatty liver or successfully reduced liver inflammation can be highly motivating. Whether through in-person groups or online forums, sharing experiences can offer new ideas and a sense of accountability. These connections remind you that you are not navigating the journey alone.

Social support also helps in navigating environments that are not always health-focused. Having people around who respect your choices makes it easier to decline foods or habits that could hinder liver regeneration. It also creates opportunities to enjoy shared activities that align with your health goals, such as cooking classes, farmers' market trips, or group exercise.

As your habits solidify and your health continues to improve, your own story can become a source of encouragement for others. Sharing what you have learned and the changes you have made not only reinforces your own commitment but also contributes to a wider awareness about the importance of liver health.

Get Your Free E-book

Get Your Free E-book
Scan the QR code below to instantly access the e-book ‘ **The Liver-Cleanse Pantry**’, absolutely free

SCAN ME

https://bonus.grapevinebooks.com/livercleansepantry